the great fitness experiment

the great fitness experiment

ONE • YEAR • OF • TRYING • EVERYTHING

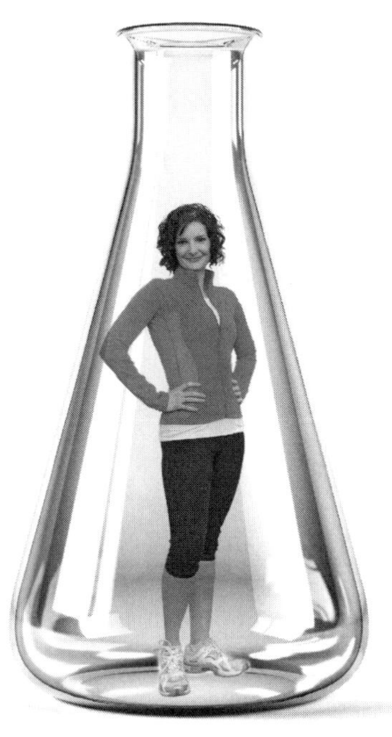

by

Charlotte **H**ilton **A**ndersen

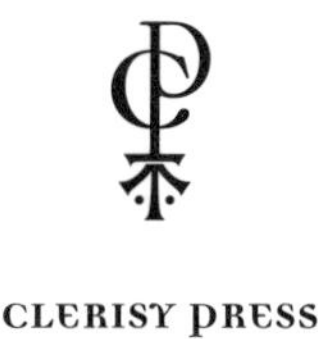

CLERISY PRESS

The Great Fitness Experiment

Published by Clerisy Press
Printed in the United States of America
Distributed by Publishers Group West
First edition, first printing

For further information, contact the publisher at:
Clerisy Press
PO Box 8874
Cincinnati, OH 45208-08074
www.clerisypress.com

Library of Congress Cataloging-in-Publication Data
Andersen, Charlotte Hilton.
The great fitness experiment : one year of trying everything / by Charlotte Hilton Andersen.
p. cm.
Includes bibliographical references.
ISBN-13: 978-1-57860-475-3
ISBN-10: 1-57860-475-3
1. Physical fitness. I. Title.
RA781.A592 2011
613.7—dc22

2010032793

Edited by Donna Poehner
Cover designed by Stephen Sullivan
Text designed by Annie Long
Photos courtesy of the author

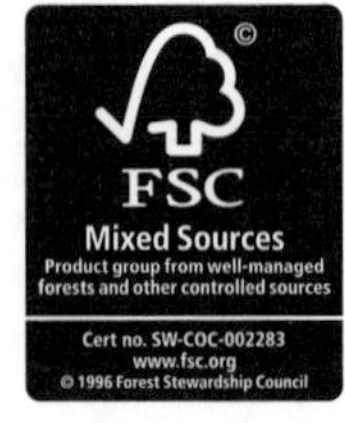

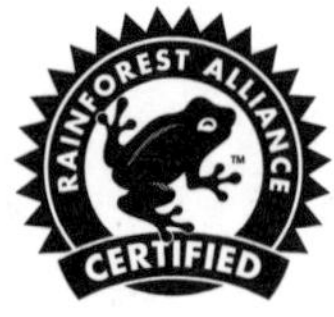

Table *of* Contents

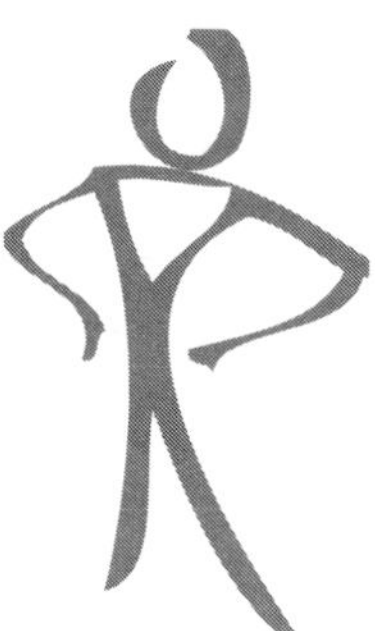

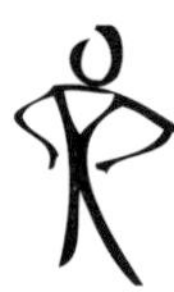

To my love, Jason, my children, my family, and
my gym buddies Allison, Megan, and Krista:
Thank you for all your love, support, and unfailing patience.
You are what makes doing this fun!

the great fitness experiment

Introduction

I GET ASKED A LOT OF QUESTIONS WHEN PEOPLE HEAR my life's pursuit is trying out every fitness program on the planet. Lots of them involve some permutation of "Are you crazy?" (Answer: Yes, and in more ways than you know.) Or "Why does eating an eight-ounce chocolate bar make me gain three pounds?" (Answer: Because Weight Watchers and Hershey's are in cahoots—it's a global conspiracy. Seriously, I have no idea; the physics don't make sense to me either.) But the single question I hear most often is: "So, what is the best way to eat and exercise?"

As if I would actually give you that answer right in the introduction of my book and thereby allow you to skip reading the rest of my hilarious and insane antics! If I were a real fitness professional, I'd make you wade through pages of randomly **BOLDED** and **CAPITALIZED** stuff with lots of extraneous punctuation!!! and hyperbolic promises (You WILL get the RIPPED BODY of your dreams in just 25.2 days by just changing your thought patterns!?!?! Oh, and maybe doing some crack.) And don't forget the random-yet-oddly-compelling testimonials from people you've never met but have now seen in a G-string and a fake tan. Thank goodness for you, I'm not professional!

Here it is: The best exercise and nutrition program out there is . . . pretty much all of them. It turns out that anything that has you eat less crap and move more will get you results. It's not glamorous but it's true. The problem is not that you haven't found the One Perfect Program yet; the problem is that you're not asking the right questions. Let me help you out.

Q: *Which fitness program will get me the biggest results in the shortest amount of time?*

a: Anything with a lot of high intensity interval training combined with very heavy weight lifting. CrossFit (chapter 3) will grow you some serious muscle in as little as a month. Be ready to pay for your results with a lot of pain though. These workouts are not for the faint of heart or weak of stomach. They are also not for people just beginning to get into fitness. These programs will knock you flat on your back until you see stars, and they won't even buy you dinner first.

Q: *Which fitness program is best for a beginner?*

a: Whichever one you can stick with! Ideally, you'd do some mix of cardio and weight training—The Monkey Bar Gym Workout (chapter 1) is a great place to start if you'd like a specific recommendation—but if you don't love it, you probably won't continue to do it. And with exercise, simply showing up is 90 percent of the battle. So dance; rock climb; kickbox, play dodgeball, volleyball, or, my personal childhood favorite, "butt ball" (a game my brother and I invented, where you throw tennis balls at each other's butts—we're geniuses, I know)—just so long as you keep moving. You can add in the other stuff once you get addicted to the endorphin rush.

Q: *Which fitness program is the best for home workouts?*

a: While the late-night ShamWow gurus (I'm allowed to make fun of the ShamWow guy now that he's done a stint in prison, right?) would have you believe that you will never be able to get a tight, toned midsection or a good cardio burn without their gadgetry, the truth is there are a lot of great workouts you can do with very minimal equipment (see the TRX in chapter 8) or even with just bodyweight alone (see the Celebrity Workout in chapter 4). Plus you spare yourself the embarrassment factor of being betrayed by your own bodily fluids in a very public place. (And, yes, I realize that the ShamWow is not technically a fitness tool, but you could use it as one—see the Action Hero Workout in chapter 5.)

Q: *Which fitness programs can I take with me to the gym?*

a: All of them! While most workouts can be adapted for home use, you will have more options at a gym—more options for exercise and also more options for fun. Fortunately for you and all the people who work out at my YMCA, I am not easily embarrassed. Despite having humiliated myself in nearly every way possible (Split my pants? Check! Pinned myself down with a weighted bar? Check! Fallen off the treadmill, the stair climber, the arc trainer and even regular nonmoving stairs? Check, check, and double check!) I adore working out in the gym and have managed to adapt every workout to be able to be done there. Really it's all about the free childcare and not my narcissistic need for attention, I swear.

Q: *Which workout will help me drop weight the fastest?*

a: None of them. Here's a little-told truth in the fitness industry: exercise makes you hungry. Don't get me wrong, I am not telling you to quit exercising! Exercise is good for you on so many levels. Everything from your mind to your mood to your newly lifted butt cheeks will benefit from a good sweat fest, but all of your weight loss is going to happen in the kitchen. Most professionals I've talked to say weight loss is about 70 percent nutrition and 30 percent exercise. For me, those proportions are closer to 85/15. It takes me five minutes to eat a baggie of jelly beans (yes, I wrote "baggie"—I package my high fructose corn syrup up like crack, it's that addictive) but an hour of kickboxing to burn those suckers off. Do the math and you'll see that watching what you eat will give you scale results a lot faster than exercise alone. Don't drop the exercise, but at the same time don't kid yourself that just because you did an hour Spin class you can eat whatever you want the rest of the day. Unless you are Michael Phelps—and then carry on, sir. You and your nuclear metabolism are a national treasure.

Q: *Which workout is the worst?*

a: Well I avoid the obviously idiotic ones—chin presser thingy anyone? But I have done some fitness programs that my body has not responded well to at all and have ended in spectacular failure (see The Primal Blueprint, chapter 7). This is where the "Experiment" part of The Great Fitness Experiment comes in. People's bodies react differently to different diet and exercise plans. This journey was all about finding what worked and didn't work for me. If it helps you too or at least gives you a good laugh (you can count that as an ab workout!), then my work here is done.

Q: *Who are you to tell me how to work out?*

a: I want to be the first to tell you that while I hold two degrees—a Bachelor's of Science in Psychology and a Master's of Science in Computer Information Systems—they are completely irrelevant to health and fitness. I'm no expert. My Experiments are not scientifically rigorous. Basically, I'm just a girl trying to get a good workout in and making a lot of mistakes along the way. For added fun and to get some additional perspective, I have managed to rope in a fair number of talented, smart, and hilarious people to do the Experiments with me, both in the gym and online. My hope is that this will inspire you to try some new things and find a way to sweat that you truly love (and that won't get you a ticket for indecent behavior).

Q: *Can you share any tricks you've discovered?*

a: Just one: Get a support system. If there is one thing I have learned, it is that people exercise more and at a greater intensity—not to mention have a lot more fun—when they do it with a friend or five. Even if you are the type who would rather hit the trail with naught but Miley Cyrus chirruping in your ear (don't worry, I never judge a person by their taste in workout tunage—your secret is safe with me!), at least have someone you check in with to stay accountable and share war stories. In this book you will meet many of my Gym Buddies, like Allison, the only Gym Buddy who has been with me through every single Experiment and whom we liken to She-Ra for how amazingly strong she is; and Megan, who has run a marathon and also cracks the best inappropriate jokes; and Krista, the only Gym Buddy who genuinely enjoys handstand pushups. Then there are the instructors like Turbo Jennie, who teaches a wildly popular TurboKick kickboxing class and will call you if you miss a class; or Bootcamp Bill, who let me Experiment on his class; or Trainer Jim, who has taken my body fat percentage so many times that he knows my stretch marks better than I do. I'm also very blessed to have a loyal band of readers on my Web site who support and laugh at, and, when necessary, chide me on a daily basis. Remember, you are working to build a lifelong love of exercise, and surrounding yourself with people you love and who love you will ensure that you not only keep at it but that you also enjoy it.

THROUGH DOING THE GREAT FITNESS EXPERIMENT on my Web site for nearly three years now, I have discovered what my life's purpose is: to be a cautionary tale to others. So sit back, enjoy the ride, and hopefully you'll learn a few things—even if it's just that you're glad you're not me!

Author's note: These Experiments were done mostly in 2007. At the time, I had three boys, the youngest being just a few months old and still nursing. I began my first Experiment in October of 2006 and completed my last Experiment chronicled in this book in September of 2007. Since then I have added a daughter and three more years of fitness experimenting fun.

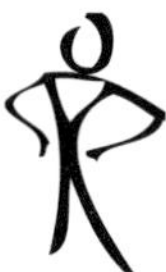

chapter one

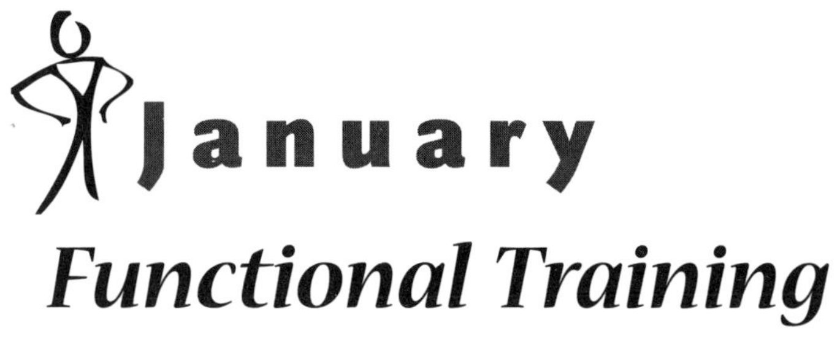

January
Functional Training

PEOPLE WILL ASK YOU A LOT OF STRANGE QUESTIONS while you are hanging upside down by your knees from a chin-up bar. Perhaps the position makes you look approachable. Or maybe it's just because they enjoy the power of knowing they can reach out and poke you in the ribs and make you crash on your head if the yen strikes them. I've had a stockbroker—who I'd never met right-side up—tell me that he cheats on his taxes and then ask me if I thought that was a conflict of interest. (Conflict of interest? No. Conflicted morals? Absolutely.) I've had a mother tell me she thinks the Jonas Brothers are hot and then asked me if that makes her a pervert. (Confession: I've checked out The Wiggles on several occasions, and I don't mean at the library.) But the question I get most often from strangers meandering by me on the weight floor is some variation of "What on earth are you doing?"

My reply, whether I'm hanging by my knees, doing handstands in the corner, or cartwheels across the floor, is, "When's the last time you saw a kid working out?" Now, in this day of pint-sized elliptical machines and Spin classes for middle schoolers, the answer is a little murky, but if you let a child just do what they want, they don't work out. They *play out*. And, according to the proponents of functional fitness in general and Jon Hinds of the Monkey Bar Gym (www.monkeybargym.com) in particular, that's what we should be doing as well. Not only is it more fun, but you get a better workout in a shorter amount of time.

The Theory

WEIGHT MACHINES ARE FOR LOSERS. And I'm not talking weight loss. Those machines that take up the majority of gym real estate are for people who want to lose muscle, joint mobility, and flexibility. Fitness, like everything, goes through fads and weight machines (like the leg press, seated military press, lat pull-down, and even the venerated Smith Machine) are definitely on their way to the "Don't" list.

This is for good reason, according to the newest fitness theory. To put it simply, you are only allowed to do the hip adductor machine if you wear knee-high socks and pull your shorts up to your bra line. (Unless, like at my gym, the adductor machine faces a huge window overlooking the basketball courts, and you love reliving your yearly visit to the gynecologist or are just an exhibitionist.)

Friends don't let friends use weight machines. But why, you say, they're easier? Exactly. And for those of you shouting, "But I've been doing them since the '80s and I loooove them." Well, then, keep on. And make sure to pump your shoes before you get started.

Weight machines help you and hurt you in the same way: They limit your natural range of motion. If you don't believe me, try a seated military shoulder press on the machine, and then try it again standing on a BOSU with free weights. I guarantee you will have to drop your weight. Want to up the ante? Try a one-legged squat with that. Unintentional bonus: You can tell people you're training to be an extra in *Karate Kid VIII,* and who doesn't love *The Karate Kid*?

Another way the weight machines hurt is that by isolating a particular muscle, they put undue strain on your joints. You may have noticed that on the leg extension machine your knees often give out before your quads. Weight machines also encourage injuries when you don't properly calibrate them to your body, thus overextending your tender ligaments. Plus, if you really have been doing them since the eighties, it's probably time for a change-up anyhow. (And lose the Zubaz pants while you're at it, please!)

Beyond slandering weight machines, functional fitness also takes on some traditional weight lifting moves, like the chest press. Despite being long revered by weight lifters as a mark of their manhood (I did actually have a date once who dropped his max press weight like Hollywood starlets name check directors), nobody actually chest presses anything in normal life. Rather, you squat, lift, push, pull, and perform a myriad of other "functional" movements.

Functional fitness exercises don't have to be limited to kiddie fare like swinging from ropes and running in circles yelling, "I'm rubber and you're glue!" Adults may prefer to work out like a nineteenth-century farmer, with moves like the axe chop and the wall throw.(What exactly is the disgruntled farmer throwing at the wall? I will leave that to your imagination. But if it meows, you've got serious psychological issues.) I love these new exercises, but I have to admit I experience a certain amount of cognitive dissonance every time I mimic pitching a bale of hay that I'm actually paying—through the wonders of modern society—to not actually have to pitch. If we still lived on subsistence farming, we'd all be getting so much "functional fitness" that gyms would go out of business. In heaven somewhere, between bites of lard-crust bacon pie, my great-great-great grandfather is rolling his eyes.

Other alternatives to traditional machine work include tried-and-true favorites like squats, lunges, medicine ball throws, and lots of free weights. If those options don't thrill you, you can always make them more difficult (and activate your core!) by standing on an unstable surface, although I feel compelled to warn you that you also up the embarrassment potential by a factor of ten.

The Workout

ALL OF THIS INFORMATION, while it made for good dinner conversation, was a little overwhelming. So for my thirty-day Experiment, I decided to use The Monkey Bar Gym program. It's free, they provide a new workout online every day, and they even have instructional videos to help you perfect your form if you haven't skip-to-my-lou'ed or chopped anything with an imaginary axe recently. All of this and more can be found on their Web site at www.monkeybargym.com

Their program is designed to be a complete workout, replacing your traditional cardio and weight routines with one comprehensive routine. This program is great because you can adjust the intensity and difficulty levels to accommodate the most beginner of fitness enthusiasts right up to seasoned athletes (in fact, Jon Hinds, the creator, is a retired professional athlete.) While the program does call for some specialized equipment, like a climbing rope, much of it can be improvised with standard gym equipment.

In the Gym

WHILE THE WORKOUTS VARY WIDELY BY THE DAY, you generally have some type of bodyweight exercises combined into a heart-pumping circuit that lasts fifteen to thirty minutes. The night before the big day I would introduce the new Experiment to the Gym Buddies (and hope none of them ran away screaming), I had to spend a solid hour on the Internet looking up the workout of the day (WOD) and then watching the videos on how to do things you think I would already know, like jumping rope.

But it all worked out for the best, as everyone was excited for three pee-inducing reasons (What? Isn't wetting yourself part of the whole return-to-childhood experience?):

1. This workout is radically different from anything else we'd ever done. Some people like doing the same old workouts over and over again, but I think most of us enjoy variety.

2. It has crazy moves like "the sea witch crawl" put into workouts like the awesome-sounding "Prison Workout." Seriously, when was the last time your workout involved anything to do with homemade tattoo guns and shivs? Fun!

3. Plus—and this may just be a bonus for me—the embarrassment, and therefore entertainment potential, is high.

So it was with much excitement that the Gym Buddies and I started our first Monkey Bar Gym WOD. It started out fun right away with several minutes of jump roping. Since we were supposed to be discovering our inner child, we skipped the boxer rope jumping. Gym Buddy Allison and I amused ourselves by reliving our second-grade jump rope champion days and showing off with double-unders, cross-overs, and split jumps. Gym Buddy Mike amused himself by mocking us. All was good fun until the inevitable happened: I snapped myself with the rope, leaving a sizeable welt that I insisted on showing to everyone despite the fact it meant I had to partially moon half the gym. I can only imagine the other half was very grateful when we moved on to the next move: the overhead carry.

Chances are good that a farmer somewhere is carrying something over his head as we speak. This fact does not make it any easier, however, to stumble your way around the track holding a forty-pound dumbbell over your head without crashing into all the senior citizens who turn to gawk. Red-faced and sweaty, we made it halfway before I wussed out and had to set the weight down. The rest of the Gym Buddies, having more upper body strength than I do, soldiered on. Instead, I set up my dumbbell like a little stool and put out my Free Advice sign. The only person who took me up on it was the Fitness Floor Manager, who asked me how I would tell someone their workout makes them look like an idiot. Good times.

Not to be discouraged, however, we finished out the workout with handstand push-ups (during which I discovered that if I close my eyes, it really feels like I'm moving up and down), jumping on and off a weight bench for several minutes (a move I can only imagine was inspired by a Spanish farmer raising bulls and did nothing to endear us to the lifters who were waiting to lie on the spot where we left our dirty footprints), and wall walks during which Gym Buddy Candice discovered she had a hole in her sock and the rest of us learned that our YMCA has a strict shoes-on policy.

You might think we would have been discouraged, but the results were truly amazing—487 calories burned in thirty minutes was only the tip of the iceberg. The next day we were sore in places we didn't know we could be sore. Plus, the welt on my butt had turned into a pretty awesome war wound. Not that I took pictures or anything. (I so totally did!)

By the halfway point, two weeks of bounding around the gym like insane people had two positive effects: a) the Gym Buddies and I had done enough WODs that our confidence and playground skills were increasing, and b) the rest of the people at our gym had gotten tired of rolling their eyes and huffing loudly and moved on to more productive cardio workouts, like running away from us whenever we came near.

In addition, we were getting stronger. Never having been able to do a pull-up before, I was enjoying the Monkey Bar way: On the playground anything goes, and so it was in this case. Any way you could get your chin over that bar counted. Jumping, swinging, frog-kicking or even standing on a Gym Buddy was all fair game. The result of all that giggling was me getting closer to doing an actual for-real pull-up than I have ever been in my post-childbearing-hips life.

The Results

JUST GOING BY THE NUMBERS, THIS is one effective workout. After just four weeks of functional training—and insane giggling—Gym Buddy Candice accomplished the nearly impossible by simultaneously losing weight (three pounds) and losing body fat (down 1 percent). Any body builder will tell you that usually you either drop body fat and maintain/gain weight (because you're

Best Moment

If you have never tried a handstand push-up, I thoroughly recommend it! Most people assume that only military folk or Cirque du Soleil freaks can manage these, but I am here to tell you that if a bunch of Minnesota mommies can manage it, you totally can. Here's a tip: Use the wall.

The first time we attempted these, we used a stairwell in front of the elevator—the only unoccupied space we could find. After we took off our shoes (no good mommy would leave marks on the wall!) and cleared a space we surveyed the wall. At first we were too scared to kick up, so we scaled it backwards like spider monkeys. Gym Buddy Allison started out the fun by closing her eyes—I have no idea why—and then after an intense moment where her face turned all purply exclaimed, "Hey, I think I'm doing it! Am I moving?" Sorry, but no.

After several weeks of practice where we finally learned how to do them with our eyes open and actually move our bodies up and down a few inches, I had the brilliant idea to attempt them without the wall. To keep my balance in the handstand position, I had to keep walking my hands. Unfortunately, I was stuck in reverse—which might have been all right had we not been in a stairwell. You can see where this is going.

I walked backwards on my hands—all the way into the elevator!

building muscle), or you drop weight but your body fat remains the same/increases slightly because of some muscle loss. It is quite a feat to do both at the same time.

Gym Buddy Allison and I had very similar results: We both maintained our weight and dropped body fat. Allison dropped an impressive 3–4 percent, and I dropped 2 percent. Gym Buddy Mike did not have his body fat tested but says he lost several pounds and that he really increased his cardio endurance. Mostly by laughing at us.

Combining the new (old?) science of functional training with high intensity intervals, this is one of the best workouts I've ever done. Besides helping all of the Gym Buddies get closer to our goals, it was also a riot. We laughed every single day. We were also sore every stinkin' day, but the laughing is definitely more important as you're more likely to stick with a workout you enjoy. I've also never had so many people interested in what I was doing. Almost every day someone asked to join us or told us it looked really fun (and hard). Another bonus is that it is an excellent calorie burn for such a short period of time—it is almost always under thirty minutes, and I burned between three hundred and six hundred calories per workout. You really can't get better than that, especially if you are time crunched.

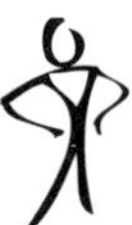

P·E·R·S·O·N·A·L | E·S·S·A·Y

How to Live to Be One Hundred (or Until the Bus Hits You)

Fiery plane crash. Rock climbing accident. Cancer. Crushed in one of those huge metal turnstiles/revolving door of spikes they have at the zoo that look like an iron maiden. (Am I the only one who is terrified by those things? I'm using the "stroller entrance" whether or not I have any kids in tow.) I wasn't sure how it was going to happen, but ever since I can remember, I've been convinced I was going to die young.

This belief has caused me to engage in some rather risky behavior (along with a severe case of political apathy—who cares who wins the election if I'm going to DIE?): cliff dancing—definitely more fun and probably more dangerous than you are imagining; meeting strangers on the Internet; scaling buildings and then jumping into dumpsters on the off chance those security cameras could make us YouTube stars; going on a week-long road trip with a guy I hardly knew (and then I married him! Hi, honey!); and a chronic habit of reading whilst walking that actually caused me to get knocked on the head by one of those mechanical arms that guard parking lots. Obviously none of these things killed me (those guard arms are lighter than they look), but that bad attitude also led me to not care overly much about my health.

Now that I am twenty-nine, I have finally come to accept the fact that I'm here to stay. And I'm very happy about that. I wake up every day grateful for my life. Things that I never gave much thought to before—pesticides, global warming, trans fats, Barack Obama, BASE jumping legality, cockroach bits in my chocolate—I suddenly have very strong and vocal opinions about. And health—mine, yours, my kids', that guy's over there—has become paramount.

So now I'm faced with the task of weeding out all those unhealthy behaviors that I ignored over the years. I've managed to get rid of the big offenders by fixing my diet, keeping up on my doctor's check-ups, exercising regularly, getting loads of therapy, and choosing *Time* over *Cosmo* in all those waiting rooms. What's left is a mish-mash of little pet neuroses.

In one of the saddest bits of research I've come across lately, the *New York Times* reports that many people avoid exercise because of severe acne. I know that other body image issues affect exercise as well. "I'm too fat to go to the gym!" "I'm too uncoordinated to play sports!" "My boobs are too big to run!" "I'd die of embarrassment if I made a mistake in step class!" "I am the six-fingered man, and there's this guy named Inigo Montoya!"

I'm not denigrating these excuses. They are definitely a source of concern, and I totally sympathize with the nagging fear that everyone is staring at your physical imperfections. But when our fears hold us back, it's time to take action.

I'm sure you've heard of the longevity study conducted by the Harvard Institute of Health. It's not terribly new. The researchers interviewed hundreds of centenarians and came up with a list of behaviors they all had in common. Note: Nowhere on the list will you find anything about being acne-free, coordinated, small-boobed, or even five-fingered.

How to Live to Be One Hundred

1. BE A GIRL. Sorry guys, it's true! Guess I *will* have the last laugh on all those horrid blind dates! Oh, wait, I already do.

2. HAVE GOOD GENES. Another one you can't choose but stick around because the rest of the list is all stuff under your direct control.

3. ENGAGE IN A GREAT DEAL OF PHYSICAL ACTIVITY. See? Doesn't matter if you punch yourself in the face in boxing—which I have totally done btw—all that matters is you are movin' and groovin'.

4. EAT LITTLE OR NO MEAT. I didn't make that up. It's in there, I swear!

5. DON'T SMOKE. If you do, stop.

6. DON'T DRINK HEAVILY.

7. GAIN LITTLE TO NO WEIGHT IN ADULTHOOD. Easier said than done, Harvard!

8. DON'T OVEREAT. The famously long-lived Okinawans in the study took in about 10-20 percent fewer calories than the average American adult. They actually have a philosophy: Eat until you are 80 percent full. When you figure out how to tell when you hit that 80 percent mark, please let me know.

9. CONSUME LESS FAT and make the fat you do eat of the good variety (nuts, fish, Chris Farley.)

10. EAT LOTS OF FRUITS AND VEGGIES.

11. GET REGULAR PHYSICAL ACTIVITY AS LONG AS YOU ARE ABLE.

12. CHALLENGE YOUR MIND.

13. HAVE A POSITIVE OUTLOOK.

14. MAINTAIN CLOSE TIES WITH FAMILY AND FRIENDS.

The researchers conclude by saying that no matter what our gender or our genes predispose us to, most of us could add a decade or more to our lives simply by doing the above things. So if you, like me, have finally decided that the universe is not out to get you, try making a few tweaks. Start with the last one, it'll make you feel better almost instantaneously. Plus, your mom called. She wants to tell you she loves you. And then she wants to do the I-told-you-so dance because, really, she *was* right about the peas.

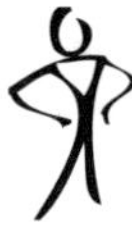

chapter two

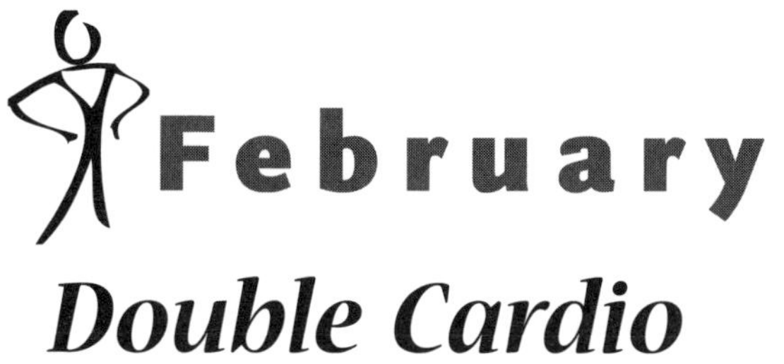

February

Double Cardio

"If one day, by some freak chance, I were to wake up fat, then I would do double cardio every day until I wasn't."

~ Tom Venuto, professional body builder and author of *Burn the Fat, Feed the Muscle,* explaining the body builder's secret to rapid fat loss.

The Theory

IF SOME IS GOOD, MORE IS ALWAYS BETTER. Right? Money, chocolate, sex, success, even thinness—our society tells us to always go for more. Right away I'm assuming you can see the flaw to this logic. That's because you have common sense. Me, I've never met a problem I didn't think couldn't be solved by just trying harder. And so when I found myself carrying some extra weight after popping out five kids in seven years, I decided to lose those last eight pounds, kamikaze style.

Up to that point in my life, most of my fitness instruction had come from body builders. I mean, seriously, look at those people—if there's one thing they know how to do, it's lose fat and gain muscle. (Okay, that and tan. You know you're a body builder when you are forced to go online to buy self tanner because the store doesn't carry anything dark enough for your tastes.) In addition to reading all the greats: Bill Pearl, Tom Venuto, Rippetoe, and even the mighty Ahnold (as in Schwarzenegger), I also read a lot of fitness magazines and Web sites. The general consensus, even supported by reputable institutions like the American Diabetes Association, was that while building muscle was good, cardio was the ultimate fat burner.

I latched on to Tom Venuto's statement like a lifeline and went to work designing my ultimate cardio plan. Incidentally, I don't blame Tom for what happened next. He's a smart cookie and can't be held accountable for my predilection for extreme behavior. One look at the guy—he has abs so washboard that real washboards (do those still exist?) cry in shame—and you can tell that what he does obviously works. For him. I like an extreme mindset. I love extreme results.

The Workout

Since I was already in the gym five days a week doing cardio with three of those workouts followed by weights, I didn't want to take any more time away from my kids, so I knew I was going to have to get creative to fit in a second workout. I decided to take up running. At night. In the dark. In the winter. When I couldn't handle the minus-forty-degree temps anymore (I do live in Minnesota, state motto: Your Boogers Will Freeze Your Nose Shut), I'd head to the gym at o-dark-thirty before my husband went to work. I'd take the kids to the park and run laps around the perimeter with my baby in the stroller. As a last resort, I'd do videos while the kids napped. It wasn't easy at first, but eventually I settled in to the new schedule. I figured I only had to keep up this insanity until I lost those pesky eight pounds, and then I'd drop back to a more reasonable "maintenance" schedule.

In the Gym

AT NO POINT DID I THINK my burgeoning obsession with those eight pounds was abnormal. Sure, I worked out more than most people, but that's what *I do*. Fitness is my hobby, my passion, my love, my . . . whole life?

After two months of this schedule, the scale hadn't budged. Ever the optimist, I thought perhaps I had gained some muscle mass and headed into the gym to get my body fat tested. I had gained 2 percent body fat. I am not proud of this: I went down Lindsay Lohan style, rolling around on the floor and crying until the personal trainer fled, fearing his own safety. How could I have worked so hard for the past two months and then gained body fat? (It should be noted that as my weight had stayed the same, what was actually happening was that I was losing muscle as my body was burning it to fuel my long cardio sessions.)

One would think that at this point I would realize that my Experiment was a failure and call it quits. And possibly get help for what was subtly but surely becoming an eating disorder in the form of compulsive exercise. Sadly, that realization wouldn't hit for many more months. Instead, I decided that if the cardio wasn't working it was because I was simply eating too much. As a nursing mother working out heavily twice a day, you'd think if anyone would get to eat whatever she wanted, it would be me. Rather than enjoy my gustatory freedom, I instead fixated on those stupid eight pounds and cut one hundred calories a day. Then two hundred. Then five hundred. Finally, I lopped eight hundred calories off. Surely this would work!

Two more months of this madness, and the scale actually started to creep up on me. You'd think that my highly honed skills of observation would have made me realize at this point that my experiment wasn't working, and I needed to do something else. After all, it was Einstein (or possibly Ben Franklin or Mark Twain—heck, even Dr. Phil jumped on this train) who said, "The definition of insanity is doing the same thing over and over and expecting different results." You would be underestimating the amount that I really wanted this to work.

I knew I was losing precious muscle, so I figured I should add some more weight lifting. I upped the ante from three days a week to five. And I kept the double cardio because I was afraid that if I stopped at this point, I'd gain even more weight. I lasted two more months (bringing me to a grand insane total of six months of double cardio) before my body decided to give out on me.

Out of the Gym

I GOT A STRESS FRACTURE IN MY RIGHT SHIN. All the exercise combined with undernourishment, plus the demands of nursing a baby, made my body go kaput. At first I went nearly wild when the doctor told me what had happened. And not because of the pain—which was pretty bad; I couldn't even walk up stairs or flex my toes without tears coming to my eyes—but because that meant I couldn't do my cardio. I couldn't run. I couldn't kickbox. I couldn't do step aerobics or BOSU or even regular floor aerobics. The treadmill was dead to me.

The doctor advised me to take four weeks off of all exercise and six-to-eight weeks off weight-bearing exercise. After icing my shins (now the left one was starting to hurt too), the next day I was back in the gym, on the stationary bike. My friends applauded what they saw as my tenacity and flexibility, but after running three miles on the treadmill, just praying for the pain to go away, I was finally beginning to realize that I had a problem that went way beyond a hairline fracture in my tibia.

It hadn't worked. I hadn't lost the weight, but I sure had lost my mind. It was then I finally came across some emerging research about cardio. After looking back through my pages of notes—every day I write down my workout, calories burned, weight and body fat percentage, (yep, I am that neurotic!)—I came to a head-smacking realization. The longer and harder I worked out, the more weight and fat I gained. The less I worked out, the more my weight dropped or remained the same.

This goes against everything we're told about exercise, particularly in regards to cardio being the Almighty Fat Burner. The American Heart Association officially recommends thirty-to-sixty minutes of cardio per day for weight maintenance and sixty-plus minutes per day for weight loss. According to this, I should have been losing weight by the bucket. And yet, my results were not consistent with this.

It turns out that my Case of the Creeping Poundage was not totally without precedent. As I poked around on Internet fitness discussion groups and talked to other women in my running group, I came across a phenomenon called "the marathon effect." I discovered that many runners experience weight gain when they up their mileage—even into the elite levels. Mark Sisson, a former professional Ironman and author of *The Primal Blueprint* (see July's chapter for more on that Experiment), writes, "Intense Cardio (long stretches of a sustained 80 percent of max heart rate) raises cortisol levels, increases oxidative damage, systemic inflammation, depresses the immune system, and decreases fat metabolism."

He recommends (and practices) a few days a week of low-to-moderate intensity cardio (like brisk walking) with one-to-two days a week of short, very high-intensity interval sprints (he sprints for twenty-to-forty seconds, then rests and repeats four-to-eight times). Finally, he adds three days a week of weight lifting. This workout would be substantially less than what I was doing.

There is another factor in weight gain besides exercise, of course: nutrition. Everyone knows that the more energy you expend in exercise, the more energy your body will take in in fuel. But what that means in reality is that exercise makes you hungrier. It's a major "duh," and yet I had never made the connection between my long runs and my crazy hunger afterward.

Actress Courtney Thorne-Smith said in an interview with *Fit Pregnancy* magazine, "I used to run eight miles a day, then go to the gym, do weights and then yoga, until I realized that I was so hungry and tired all the time. So I stopped doing all that and started just walking. I feel so much freedom now: I don't have to stay in a hotel with a gym, and I'm never so hungry that I panic. A lot of women are in a crazy exercise cycle; they're so afraid they'll gain weight if they stop. What they need to realize is that if you're not exercising so much, you don't have to eat so much, and your body adjusts. It sounds so simple, but you really do have to listen to your body."

I can count the number of times on one unmanicured hand that something a celebrity has said really hit home to me, but this statement was the bucket of ice poured over my head that I needed.

I realized that for me, long stretches of high-intensity exercise also increase cravings for sugar. Which would make sense, considering the huge sports supplement industry making gels, gus (grown-up sodas), and carb drinks (all of which are straight sugar) for runners and cyclists. I began to notice that when I got home from a really intense workout, I would be shaky and weak and nauseous—symptoms that only passed after I threw back a handful of gummy worms. It's funny, the craving would be so intense that I'd eat things that I normally don't ever enjoy, like marshmallows, circus peanuts, or even plain sugar on a spoon. The days I exercised less, it seemed my cravings were easier to control.

The Results

Too much exercise is bad. No exercise is also bad. It was time for this extreme girl to find herself some moderation. (But I'm soooo bad at moderation!) I wasn't ready to follow Mark Sisson's and Courtney Thorne-Smith's advice and drop all my endurance workouts, but I knew I had to cut back. I finally stopped the double cardio. I dropped the weight sessions back to every other day. But the biggest change came when I discovered Tabata intervals, a form of high-intensity interval training.

Due to the shin fracture, I was still limited as to what types of exercise I could do, and so I returned to the short HIIT intervals on the bike as explained in Chapter 10. My sugar cravings mostly went away, my shins felt better, and within one month I'd lost 1.5 percent body fat and three pounds.

Conclusions

It isn't often that my Great Fitness Experiments are utter failures. The fact is that any exercise can work for you, and often it is just the change itself that will produce results, so generally every workout I try has some positive results. Not double cardio. I feel it is very important to talk about my Great Fitness Failure

Worst Moment

My third son, nine months old at the time, was in the hospital fighting a terrible infection that required IV antibiotics. I spent two straight days holding his feverish body while he was poked and prodded; the only way he would sleep was if I were standing and rocking him. After watching twenty-four hours of Home and Garden Television in such a state of bleary-eyed exhaustion that painting my kitchen chartreuse actually seemed like a good plan, my husband came to spell me so I could go home, take a shower, and get some sleep for a couple of hours. What did I do as soon as he got there? I drove straight to the gym and did a kickboxing class followed by an hour of running—in my street clothes because I didn't have any gym clothes handy, and I didn't want to waste any time going home to get them. Because I couldn't miss a workout. Not when I was sick. And not even when my precious baby was sick. Even then I wasn't yet willing to admit I had a problem with compulsive over-exercising. I have done a lot of stupid things as a mother (yes, I've already established a therapy fund for my children), but this was my lowest point. I cried all the way back to the hospital, and yet I couldn't stop myself.

as the more-is-better approach is a trap that a lot of exercisers fall into. Not only does it lead to painful conclusions like broken bones and "overtraining syndrome"—a syndrome I later had another brush with when I ended up with a suppressed thyroid from over-exercising—but it takes a great toll mentally. We hear a lot about the eating disorders anorexia and bulimia, but compulsive over-exercising (and binge eating for that matter) are rarely talked about despite being as detrimental to one's health and sanity.

It's been two-and-a-half years since my Double Cardio Experiment, and it's been a roller coaster. First, the bad news: I'm still working out twelve-to-fifteen hours a week. For comparison, my therapist (you knew I would have one by this point, right?) would like me to keep it under ten. The American Heart Association recommends three hours a week for basic health maintenance.

But now the good news! At least I'm down from the twenty-five hours a week I was working out. But wait, there's more—I've also taken down the intensity level of several of my workouts. Rather than try and push it for the whole two hours I'm at the gym, I now do my scheduled workout and then use the extra time to just walk the track or stretch with a Gym Buddy or two and catch up on the status of all the celebrity wombs. And this last tidbit may fall under the umbrella of too much information, but as it is a good indicator of my overall health, I feel inclined to share. My periods have finally come back and are now on a regular schedule! (Strange side note: Weirdly, my cycle has synched up with Turbo Jennie and Gym Buddy Sunny. I never get to be the alpha female! Ah well, I'll send them the bill for my chocolate cravings and zit cream.)

P·E·R·S·O·N·A·L | E·S·S·A·Y

Confessions of a Compulsive Over-Exerciser

Most people have a hard time getting to the gym. I have a hard time getting out of the gym. My love of everything fitness has become my defining personality trait. That is often what people know me for. It doesn't help that my hobbies include reading about fitness, writing about fitness, and talking about fitness. And don't forget, you know, actually exercising.

In a country where two-thirds of the population is overweight and two-thirds of the starlets are underweight, someone who is very committed to their exercise regimen is often seen as smart, dedicated, energetic, and principled. Which I hope that I am. However, I am also crazy.

That is not a word my therapist likes—and I mention my therapist here at the outset so all of you will relax in the knowledge that I am "getting help"—but crazy is a pretty apt descriptor of my mental state. I am a person of extremes. A perfectionist. A black-and-white thinker. Type A personality. Call it what you want, but what it all boils down to is being bad at balance.

This pattern of extreme positions has been replayed many times over in my life. My passion is often what draws people to me, and my fanaticism is what drives them away. With me, it's two sides of the same coin. On one hand, I was a straight A student, valedictorian of every graduating class I've ever been in. On the other hand, I can be a ferocious know-it-all despite my glaring ignorance in many subjects. And then there's the food. On one hand, I am very educated on health and healthy eating. On the other hand, I was so eating disordered that we had to make up a name—orthorexia—to accurately describe all my neuroses about food (see chapter 11). All of which brings me to exercise. First anorexic, then orthorexic, and now—ta da!—compulsive exerciser.

What Makes an Exercise Addict?

Athletes work out eight-to-twelve hours a day, and nobody calls them exercise bulimics. Usually. So what makes an exercise addict? First, it's not just about the time spent exercising, although that can be a good starting point. Just like a person who fasts for religious purposes is not generally an anorexic, not all people who exercise a lot are addicts. For me, the difference is in the mindset.

1. THE GOALS. Athletes work out to train for a sport or event. If something in their training causes injury or is not furthering their goals, they stop doing it. A compulsive exerciser will work out regardless of the consequences. They may have performance goals, but, sadly, they usually go no further than the oblique and unattainable "to be thinner" or "to run faster" or "to build endurance" or "to lose body fat." Injuries are something to be tolerated and worked through as taking a break from exercising feels impossible.

2. THE BREAKS. An athlete will put 100 percent of their focus into training, but once a goal is accomplished they can take a break. Often their breaks are built into their training schedule—a technique called periodization, meant to maximize gains while sparing the body. Take Michael Phelps, for example. In a 2008 interview with *Outside* magazine, the interviewer chides him for gaining weight (stupid interviewer), and Michael responds very sanely with something along the lines of: "Whatever. I just swept the freaking Olympics. I can take a break. I start training for the 2012 Olympics in 2009, so I'm just going to enjoy myself right now." (Concerns about enjoying himself with a bong, duly noted.) For a compulsive exerciser, the result is the exercise—or the release of anxiety they get from the exercise—and so the score resets to zero every day. It doesn't matter what you did yesterday or what you have scheduled tomorrow, you feel compelled to workout at 100 percent every single day. The voices in your head just won't shut up until you do.

3. THE RESULTS. An athlete is all about the results. Did I get a better time? Win the medal? Ace my opponent? For a compulsive exerciser, the results are often more in the form of overuse injuries—stress fractures and bad knees and sore elbows that are never quite allowed to heal. This can be compounded by the fact that over-exercising often goes hand in hand with under-eating. What over-exercisers often do not realize (or choose to ignore) is that exercising too much will not get you where you want to be. After a certain point, exercise actually has the reverse effect on your body, causing you to gain weight and body fat because of the constant stress you are putting it under. Not to mention you are jeopardizing your long-term health by weakening your bones, damaging your heart (it's a muscle, after all), and even wrecking your fertility.

How Did I Get Here?

So, besides being just generally compulsive, how does one become an exercise addict? Well, it's quite simple. I have valid reasons why I exercise. Feeling strong, safe, and sane are very compelling—and legitimate—reasons to seek out that endorphin rush. But other motivations have crept in over the years. I believe it is these other motivators, primarily based out of fear, that have pushed me over the edge from "girl who likes to exercise" to "crazy girl who over-exercises."

FEAR OF HUNGER. Exercise is my permission to eat. I'm not actively eating disordered now, but part of that is because I feel like I've earned the right to eat because I've exercised. No exercise? My mind says no food. I don't starve, but that's only because I never miss a workout. In addition, I am terrified of feeling hungry. I am so afraid that if I just let myself eat, I'll eat anything and everything, and I'll never stop. But as long as I'm exercising, I'm not hungry. (What happens in the thirty minutes after a really intense workout is an entirely different story.)

FEAR OF FAT. I am particularly ashamed of this feeling because it shows how entirely I've bought into our society's perception of fat = evil. Even though rationally I know it isn't true, it still lurks in the back of my mind. See, I think that there are people for whom being thin is a natural state, and then there are people for whom being thin takes a lot of hard work and constant vigilance. I am of the latter variety. Whether or not it is true, I believe that I hold my body at a weight that it would not choose, if left to its own devices.

FEAR OF ANXIETY. This is probably the reason that holds the most power for me. I use exercise as my stress reliever. I'm a very anxious person, and exercise—intense exercise—is the quickest way to feel better. Unfortunately, a lot of anxiety requires a lot of exercise to burn it off. Those of you who have been through Psych 101 will recognize this as the classic OCD cycle.

FEAR OF MYSELF. I often tell people that the only time I like me is when I'm working out. It is a sad statement, and I am working on changing that, but at the moment it is true. The only time when I am not harshly critical of my body is when I'm exercising. There—in the gym—is when I am proud of it for everything it can do, when I stop punishing it for feeling hungry or for my chubby thighs, when I allow it to feel sexy and smart. If only I could hold onto that feeling, but it fades as quickly as my runner's high.

IT'S ADDICTING. Anyone who has hit that place of euphoria that you can only reach from intense physical exertion knows that your first thought afterward is, "How can I get back here?" I'm an adrenaline junkie.

The Problem with Compulsive Exercise

Despite its reputation for being the disorder that everyone wishes they had, there are many downsides to compulsive exercise. First, it's very time consuming. If left on my own, I'll work out upwards of five or six hours a day. However, thanks to my children, I am never left on my own, which becomes self limiting. Second, it often has the opposite of the desired effect. I first took up running to lose weight. But as you just read, I've discovered that if I run too much, I actually gain weight. Third, I've experienced many negative health effects resulting from over-training, like amenorrhea, a suppressed thyroid, and a myriad of smaller injuries. The greatest toll, however, is on my mind. By making my self-worth dependent on something so capricious as a good workout, I've set myself up for a veritable roller coaster of highs and lows.

Learning to Balance

I have to admit, it's hard to talk about this. In a way, I feel like it reduces my credibility. But in the end I feel like it's more important to speak the truth about my experiences as well as my Experiments. So it's probably going to be all right. By this point, I am sure some of you are nodding your heads as well. If I've learned one thing from talking and writing extensively on this subject it's that I know I'm not the only compulsive exerciser out there.

Other People's Stories

My exercise addiction is probably the topic I get the most e-mails about from my Web site. Most people are just curious or want to offer support, but there are always a few who can relate only too well. I'd like to share with you two e-mails I have received from readers recently that typify exactly what I am talking about. I think many of you may see yourself in them. I know I did. Both of these letters I could have written myself at different points in my life. Reader K (letters have been changed to protect the alphabet) represents the extreme end of the spectrum. She writes:

I'm a twenty-one-year-old college senior and maybe I seem successful; I'm fit and talented at my craft (illustration, which is my major, and all of my teachers told me I am among the best in my class) and highly driven in work and school (grades came out straight A's) and I'm told often I'm attractive.

But I have no social life to speak of because it would interfere with my exercising (which, frankly, would consume my entire day were it not for my classes, school work, and job that make me appear a semi-normal human being). Also, people think the way I eat is weird, which is true because I've been eating disordered for over half my life now.

This escapes most people's attention because I eat healthy most of the time (with obsessive strictness to vitamin, protein, fiber, and fat intake) and exercise (which in most people's minds equals "healthy" and admirable even though it is taken to extreme).

My BMI dances between 16 and 15.8, depending on the day. I have not had a period in almost a year. I have 11 percent body fat and a lot of lean muscle; in short, I currently have the body make-up of a twelve-year-old boy. I have no hobbies anymore that do not involve fitness and nutrition. I check mirrors when no one is looking to check my fat and flex my muscles, out of the fear they will disappear should I neglect to exercise for a day (which I can't bring myself to do).

For a while, I have been content with this obsession, but I feel I need to make changes for the better and soon before something really bad happens (I've been lucky enough that even at my stupidest, a forty-mile bike trip on just nine hundred calories that day, I didn't collapse with a heart attack) and ruins everything I've ever worked for that matters.

Reader B is a really good example of how compulsive exercising starts out and how insidious it can be. She writes:

Just today I read your entry about being a compulsive over-exerciser, and it was (sadly) an "Aha!" moment for me. I so saw myself in your description of yourself, and I finally realized (I may be the last person who knows me to do so) that yeah, I may just have a problem! What's scary is that I was so deluded and telling myself it was healthy healthy healthy while simultaneously being somewhat secretive about it so that no one would judge me or try to stop me. And coming up with creative ways to "sneak in" working out. And happily looking at my little log of activities and calories burned for the day. And fantasizing about having the freedom to work out all day like a professional athlete. And excitedly drawing up and continuously tweaking my training schedule. And on and on . . .

I'm not sure how bad all of these things are by themselves. But when you are working out one-to-three hours per day and wishing it was more, well—it may be time to reassess, eh?

My Advice

If you think that you suffer from compulsive over-exercising, you need to seek help. I have a fabulous therapist and have found a lot of relief with Cognitive Behavioral Therapy (CBT). I also did a short stint on an outpatient basis through an eating disorder clinic for additional help (see chapter 5). The other key I have discovered is accountability. The Gym Buddies all know about my predilections and are not opposed to taking me aside to tell me, "Charlotte, you are looking too skinny." Or, "Charlotte, we're done with our workout. Let's just sit and stretch now." Or even, "Charlotte, you need to burn those gray pants that's how unflattering they are." In addition, I have you guys. That's why I write about this. You know I'm doing well with my compulsion when I can talk about it. If I am trying to hide it, then you have license to worry about me. The last piece of my recovery is medication. For about a year I took a combination anti-depressant and anxiolytic to help take the edge off my anxiety. I still had to deal with it by doing the work in therapy, but at least the panic wasn't so overwhelming. I'm not perfect, but I am getting better.

It is so important to realize that this is not something that is easy to change on your own. Eating disorders (and exercise bulimia is one) are pernicious! Just when I think I've got one licked, another round of craziness steps in to take its place. While it's true that I may have a more compulsive personality than most, I believe that this disorder is flourishing because society condones this particular brand of insanity. But it doesn't have to be this way. You can absolutely get better from this. You are strong. You are smart. Most importantly, you are loved. We can do this together.

chapter three

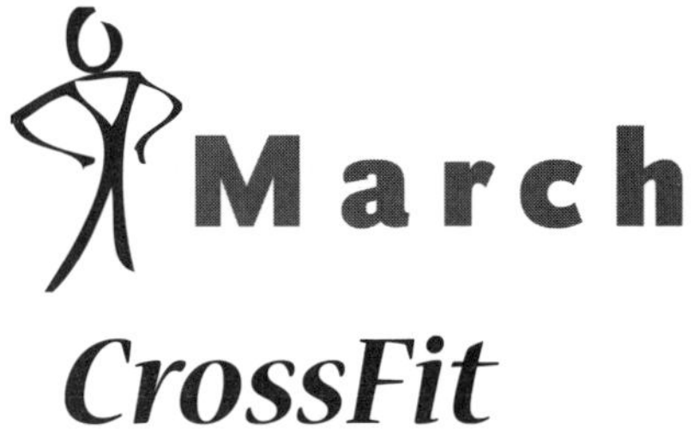

March

CrossFit

IN A DAY AND AGE WHERE "EXTREME" is printed on almost every fitness/weight-loss product (although many times it is misspelled—that's one of the lesser known side effects of diet pills; not only do they make you poor but stupid to boot), it takes a really hard-core workout to be called extreme by the world's most elite exercisers. Used by the military, police academies, and paid assassins (I'm just guessing on the last one), CrossFit is that workout.

I'm going to warn you right up front: CrossFit—as it is written—is not for beginners. Not only is it too grueling for anyone who hasn't already built a solid fitness base, but the potential for injury is high for the untrained. Danger! Intrigue! Elitism! Have I piqued your interest yet? Good. Because it is one of the best workouts I have ever tried. And once you just accept that a) it's really going to hurt, and b) you're not going to be able to do it all (at first), then it will be one of the best workouts you've ever done too. This is one workout that actually lives up to its promises of results.

The Theory

OFFICIAL CROSSFITTERS REFUSE TO BE PINNED DOWN when it comes to their workout. From the CrossFit.com Web site, CrossFit "delivers a fitness that is, by design, broad, general, and inclusive. Our specialty is not specializing. Combat, survival, many sports, and life reward this kind of fitness and, on average, punish the specialist. The CrossFit program is designed for universal scalability, making it the perfect application for any committed individual regardless of experience. We've used our same routines for elderly individuals with heart disease and cage fighters one month out from televised bouts. We scale load and intensity; we don't change programs." Yeah, they don't tell you what exactly you'll be doing; only that it is punishing and for the "committed" individual. Whether they mean committed as in dedicated or a resident of a mental facility is up for debate. My theory about this is that they are trying not to scare you off.

I'll give it to you like it is: CrossFit is scary. But in a good way. It is one the most intense, grueling, and challenging workouts you will ever try. But you can't get big results without big effort. Besides, CrossFitters are, as a group, one of the nicest, most helpful fitness communities I have ever come across. You may wet yourself, but you'll have help cleaning it up.

The Workout

CROSSFIT IS A DECEPTIVELY SIMPLE PROGRAM. Drawing elements from Olympic weight lifting, martial arts, and men's gymnastics, the keys to a CrossFit workout—called the Workout of the Day (WOD)—are high intensity and low volume. The WOD changes every day and generally combines some type of strength moves with high-intensity cardio intervals. The WOD is most often short, although occasionally they will throw in a 10K or 15K run, you know, just to keep things interesting.

CrossFit does require some equipment but nothing highly specialized; avid CrossFitters pride themselves on improvising their own home gyms. You will need first and foremost a bar on which to pull up. A weight bench, Olympic bar (forty-five pounds), and set of weight plates are also necessary. Things that are nice to have include a rope for climbing, a set of gymnastics rings, and kettlebells of various weights.

Some people choose to go to CrossFit-specific gyms that are run by certified CrossFit trainers who take care of posting the WOD and setting up all the necessary equipment. CrossFit gyms are typically very bare bones, though—no cardio machines, group fit classes, or scented eye towels—so if you sign up for one, be aware that it is a one-trick pony.

Most CrossFitters, at least in my experience, do like the Gym Buddies and I did. They go it alone or in small groups (if you come across one in a dark alley, approach slowly—they're nicer than they look but man, they're jumpy!) and make do the best they can with the limited equipment at their home or neighborhood gym. You can make it work almost anywhere, I promise you.

The actual workout is easy to follow, especially once you learn all the lingo. For instance, CrossFit kettlebell weight is given in "poods"—a Russian term that sounds dirty and while quite fun to shout across the gym floor is actually pretty benign. A pood is thirty-six pounds. Now you know. I dare you to use it in a sentence at your next dinner party. Another thing you'll need to know are the names for the various exercises. Figuring out what a muscle-up, thruster, clean and jerk, and kipping pull-up are is where the Web site is a gold mine. Not only do they have a comprehensive exercise list, but they also have some videos—set to the awesomest 80s metal ever—and other how-tos. Did I mention everything is free? Other than paying to receive the *CrossFit Journal* if you want it (and you will if you decide to go hard-core CrossFit), you don't have to pay a penny. It is a rarity in the fitness world, so enjoy it before someone figures out how to make you pay for it.

Once you get the hang of the vocabulary, all you do each day is log onto the site, write down the WOD—often named after people you probably don't know but will spend the rest of the day wondering about (who is Linda and why does she hate me so?)—and then get thee to the gym! Unless it's a surprise long run, you'll likely be done in under thirty minutes.

The Diet

CrossFitters are nothing if not comprehensive. The *CrossFit Journal* reads like a scientific dissertation on the human body, and the discussion boards are rife with theories about mitochondrial maximization and hormone cycles (it's true, men have them too!). So it only follows that they want a say over your diet. After all, even by the most generous estimates, what you do in the gym only accounts for about 30 percent of body composition. The rest is all what you put in your mouth.

CrossFit calls for a macronutrient breakdown of 30 percent protein, 40 percent carbohydrates, and 30 percent fat—i.e., The Zone ratio. Unlike The Zone diet, however, CrossFit emphasizes eating whole, natural foods and avoiding things like protein bars, frozen dinners, and the like. They also endorse the Paleolithic, or Primal, method of eating (read more in The Primal Blueprint Experiment chapter) with the main point being to limit high-glycemic carbs. For calories, they recommend setting your protein intake at 0.7–1 gram of protein per pound of lean body mass. Once you know how much protein you need, then you work the percentages backwards to figure out your total number of calories for the day. They're also fans of calorie restriction (CR), as they figure if you're crazy enough to do their workouts, then you're crazy enough to subsist on 80 percent of your calories for the rest of your life. Kidding! Actually, a lot of research has shown that CR increases longevity.

Yes, all of this requires a lot of math. First you have to find out your lean body mass (get your body fat tested, convert that percentage into pounds, and subtract that number from your total weight). Multiply that by 0.7 if you are a moderate exerciser, 1.0 if you are an athlete. Then you have to dust off the old algebra and figure out what number of calories that many grams of protein is 30 percent of. Or you can just go on the Internet. People have set up wonderfully easy-to-use calculators to help you out.

The last component of the workout is the age-old motivator competition. Each WOD is set up to allow for measurement of some kind, usually the time it takes to complete or the number of reps you can do in a certain amount of time. Upon finishing the WOD, people can go to the CrossFit.com Web site and enter in their results. Some hard-core types strive to "win" by beating the crap out of everyone else's scores. Most of us just try to beat our personal best from the last time we did that WOD. There is even a yearly CrossFit Olympics for you ultra-competitive types. Others set up CrossFit competitions in their neighborhoods or gyms. Many people find the competitive aspect highly motivating, others not so much. It's up to you how much of this you want to do—but know that it's there, if you are interested.

In the Gym

THINGS NEVER GO AS SIMPLY AS I THINK THEY WILL, and the CrossFit Experiment was no exception. After warming up and making sure we had the necessary equipment for the day, the Gym Buddies and I hit our very first WOD. It was alternating sets of clean-and-presses and clean-and-jerks. Don't know the difference? Neither did we. I'd watched the videos and still didn't really know what I was doing, but we decided to try it anyhow. That's a dangerous thing to do with CrossFit. The WOD often specifies a certain weight (like ninety-five pounds or 1.5 times your body weight), and they make no concessions for girls. Or newbies. Or weaklings. Combine ultra-heavy weights with bad form, and you have an injury waiting to happen. I almost cracked my clavicle during an aborted clean-and-press. Gym Buddy Allison was supposed to be spotting me, but since she knew as much about spotting the lift as I did about performing it, disaster ensued, and I had the bruises to prove it. Our ineptitude had a bright side though—it got the attention of Gym Buddy Mike, who just so happened to be a former college athlete and well versed in all the Olympic lifts. He took us under his wing—not literally, I love the man but he sweats like Tammy Faye Baker cries—and taught us the proper form. Who knew guardian angels pump iron? We also found out that with CrossFit, you just have to swallow your pride, start with the weight you know you can handle, and realize that their recommendations are only for people in Special Ops or possibly prison.

The next day Allison and I were back in the gym, confidence high despite the absence of Mike. The WOD was short—just five reps of three different shoulder exercises. I must admit, we were dubious. We warmed up and then went to it, doing as much weight as we could manage. It was hard. Really hard. But short! So when we finished, about fifteen minutes later, we just kinda looked at each other and shrugged. "That was . . . fun?"

And then we both bit the dust that afternoon. No joke. It didn't feel like much of a workout doing it, but that afternoon I felt like I'd run fifteen miles. I literally lay down on my (wood) kitchen floor and fell asleep while my kids ran circles around me and ate an entire box of fruit snacks. The next day I discovered that Allison had had the same crash and ended up going to bed at nine o'clock that night. It was then we discovered the phenomenon of the "metabolic reaction" so oft discussed in CrossFit circles. This mythical occurrence supposedly comes from taxing your body to its max, thereby stimulating a mass amount of human growth hormone (HGH) to be released. Your body then demands complete and total rest to build all those extra muscles it has decided you are going to need. While I have not been able to find any scientific research to back this up, the metabolic reaction seems to be a fairly typical response for newbie CrossFitters. My kids, incidentally, were thrilled and asked for a repeat performance the next day because, as my son explained it, "Go to sleep so we can eat all the potty treats again." At least he's honest. Now if only he would potty train before I have to tuck Pull-Ups into his bag when I drop him off at college.

After the metabolic reaction issue—which lessened as the month went on and our bodies got used to the rigor—the second main problem we had was with equipment. First of all, our Y only had some of the necessary equipment, and, secondly, the circuit style of most WODs leads to bad blood among other gym goers, as you either have to "claim" all the equipment in your circuit as yours or stand anxiously over them while they use it doing the weight lifter's version of the pee-pee dance. *Hurryuphurryuphurryup!*

To deal with the former problem, The Gym Buddies and I had to do a lot of improvising. Our Y considers their kettlebells proprietary equipment (not to mention they are measured in wussy pounds rather than hard-core poods), and so we had to make do with swinging regular dumbbells. Our tiny indoor track (ten laps to a mile!) is populated mainly by senior citizens with walking poles. So, often our "sprints" got caught in a traffic jam of elbows—theirs: the elderly can be surprisingly aggressive—and apologies: ours. Our "gymnastic rings" were made by hanging a TRX (see the chapter 8 on Suspension Training) from the highest beam in our gym (and sneaking the use of the janitor's ladder to do it.) And then there was the furor when we tried to make our own climbing rope by slinging two jump ropes over the chin-up bar. We might have yodeled like Tarzan too. We scared people is what I'm saying.

Fortunately, after several weeks of our shenanigans, we got a rep for being Those Crazy People, and that pretty much solved the second problem. Although, being generally polite and helpful folk, we tried to use any opportunity to recruit rather than frighten.

Out of the Gym

AS THE MONTH PASSED, I fell more and more in love with CrossFit. For one thing, it's so short that it freed up a lot of time the Gym Buddies and I could use to discuss potty training secrets, hit early garage sales (Gym Buddy Allison's greatest passion in life), or take a break in the Jacuzzi. Another awesome benefit was my new musculature. Within just a few weeks, my shoulders were noticeably stronger and, as Gym Buddy Mike pointed out one fine day, my back was so defined it "looks like a topographical map!" Which is why I was so saddened that the comment I got most frequently about our Experiment was some permutation of, "You guys are nuts! I could never do anything like that!" People were, understandably, intimidated.

What people don't realize about the Gym Buddies and me is that, other than an overabundance of crazy, we are not extraordinary athletes in any way. We are women who have birthed children. Men who work night shifts. People with old sports injuries and fears and family obligations and homework and overcrowded schedules. Our reflexes are dulled by sleepless nights from caring for our vomit-spewing spawn, our brains stunted by endless rounds of CandyLand, our nutrition curtailed by the wants of other people that we deem more important than our own. We're normal. And so I found myself repeating over and over again, "No, you don't understand! If we can do it, then you can too!" CrossFit is hard, make no mistake, but it is doable.

Charlotte's Tips for CrossFit Newbies

1. THE WOD CAN BE SCALED BACK. This is not a contest. Okay, well, technically it *is*. But that doesn't mean you have to compete! Trust me, you won't even come close to the amazons that post the top scores on the CrossFit Web site. If you can't do a pull-up (and for many people, CrossFit is where they first learn how to do a pull-up), then do a jumping pull up. Can't do that? Do negative pull-ups. Not even that? Do a nineety-degree pull-up. Still stuck to the ground? Get a wheelchair. Kidding! You can do a ninety-degree pull-up, I promise. (Position a bar in a weight rack at chest height. Crouch under the bar and grab it with both hands facing out. Pull up using as much of your arms as you can and then using your legs to help out. Start with your legs bent at a ninety-degree angle and then extend them to make it harder as you get stronger.)

If you aren't sure how to scale back the WOD, there are several Web sites that do it for you and post it every day. One to check out is BrandXmartialarts.com. CrossFitKids.com scales the WODs for children. The family that CrossFits together, stays together!

2. THE RECOMMENDED WEIGHTS ARE GOALS, NOT STARTING POINTS. Don't be me and learn this the hard way. Start small. Work up as you get comfortable.

3. PRACTICE THE LIFTS TO MAKE SURE YOUR FORM IS GOOD. If you absolutely can't/won't find a trainer to help you, then check out the CrossFit videos. Personally, I love them for the music alone. But if one of those guys shows up in a mullet, we are done. Do you hear me, CrossFit? Another good source is ExRx.net. Just type the name of the exercise into their search engine, and you'll get a video with all kinds of helpful tips. If you are a cute, young thing, then just approach the beefiest guy in the gym and ask for pointers. Show a little cleavage and you'll never have to pay for personal training again! I jest. Not that I would know this. I have no

cleavage—you all should know this by now. But please practice. Bad form will only get you injured.

4. YOU CAN REST. Most of the WODs say "AFAP" or as fast as possible. But that means as fast as is possible *for you*. Take a break if you need it. Allison and I certainly did. CrossFit WODs are built around a three-days on, one-day-off schedule. Do rest on the scheduled rest day. You've earned it!

5. WARM UP. You don't have to do the official CrossFit warm up, but you do need to get your blood moving. Run a couple of laps. Bike for five minutes. It helps.

6. KNOW YOUR LIMITS. If it starts to get overly sore, stop working that poor muscle. Like good touch/bad touch, only you can know if the pain you are feeling in your deltoid is the muscle straining to grow or just straining to detach itself from the bone. If you don't finish, you don't finish. You can always try again tomorrow.

7. THE WOD INTENSITY VARIES GREATLY. Some days are so easy that it's a little unnerving. Some days will kick you until you can't get up. And every fourth day is a rest day. So if the WOD is just too much—just know you only have to hang in there until tomorrow.

8. IF YOU ARE A BEGINNER, YOU'RE GONNA NEED A GYM. Some workouts you can modify to do at home. But unless you have an Olympic set of weights in your garage, this is a gym workout. Oh yeah, and get weight gloves. No, you won't look like a dude. Unless you are a dude. Either way, you'll thank me later.

The Results

IN WHAT I CONSIDER ONE OF THE GREATEST FITNESS COUPS of the entire year of Experimenting, CrossFit produced great, unmistakable results. In just one month. I lost a pound of weight and one percentage of body fat, which on the surface doesn't sound significant except for the fact that CrossFit changed my body *shape*. It wasn't just my shoulders that were all She-Ra Princess of Power by the end. My back, quads, biceps, and lats all showed noticeable improvement. And girls who are afraid of getting a bulky upper body? Wider shoulders make your waist look smaller! There were, however, a couple of significant downsides.

What I Liked

This workout made me feel like one seriously tough chick. It turns out I'm stronger than I thought. There is just something about heaving a huge, weighted metal bar over my head and having the entire weight floor break out in cheers and applause (what—people don't cheer at your gym?).

1. It really challenged me to up my weight. Since the WOD isn't scaled down for women, we were challenged to keep up with the men. Although we were rarely, if ever, able to do the recommended weight—215-pound deadlift, yeah right—we still lifted as heavy as we could.

2. I love that they post a new workout every day. The WOD varies in intensity and type of exercise so that over the course of a week you hit every major muscle group plus get in some intense cardio.

3. It used my competitiveness to my advantage. Seeing what everyone else posted on the Web site for their times and weight lifted really challenged me to push myself. Each day I'd report to Gym Buddies Allison, Candice, and Mike what the average was, and we would try to beat it.

4. I got to see that doing less cardio didn't hurt my fitness at all and actually probably helped me achieve my

goals better. This was a huge surprise to me. I thought I'd miss the endorphin rush of my classes, but the weight lifting provided a pretty big rush of its own and there were occasional long runs. Plus, I kept TurboKick (cardio kickboxing with a dash of hip hop flava!). Gotta get all my pent-up aggression out somehow!

5. PEOPLE THOUGHT I WAS A NUT. We got a LOT of weird looks. And yeah, that's a plus in my book. Seriously, though, this was a great community builder. People were always interested in what we were doing, and lots of people jumped in to try individual exercises or workouts.

6. BUT THE BEST PART IS THAT DESPITE LOSING VERY LITTLE WEIGHT or body fat, my upper body has seriously toned up. I can't tell you how many people have complimented me on my shoulders/biceps/back in the past couple of weeks.

What I Didn't Like

1. THE WORST PART OF CROSSFIT FOR ME wasn't the agony of a gut-wrenchingly hard workout, but rather the monotony in the range of exercises selected. They stick mainly to the Olympic lifts with heavy reliance on push-ups and pull-ups. By the end of every workout, my wrists were killing me. For a girl who makes her living typing, this was a serious issue. I also felt like my shoulders and upper back never had a chance to fully recover because we did pull-ups Every Stinkin' Day. Lots and lots of pull-ups. Hundreds of pull-ups (I'm not exaggerating; today's WOD read 125 pull-ups and 125 dips.) The most commonly lodged complaint against CrossFit across the Internet is repetitive stress injuries.

2. WE DID A LOT LESS CARDIO THAN I AM USED TO. A lot less. CrossFit only does cardio maybe once a week. And it is always running. The only variety is the distance, ranging anywhere from short sprints to 15K. If you are really, really lucky, they throw in jump roping.

3. IT'S VERY TECHNICAL. You have to make sure your form is spot on when trying to go that heavy with your weights. We would

Best Moment

The first time doing a pull-up under my own power felt like flying. Truly. I yelled and jumped around in joy. Random people clapped. It was a beautiful moment.

Also? Gym Buddy Mike told me my back musculature looked like a topographical map, which may be the nicest compliment anyone's ever given me!

have been in so much trouble without the expertise of Gym Buddy Mike. Every single one of us ended up with sore wrists, knees, or lower back. This is not a joint-friendly workout.

4. THERE IS A LOT OF POTENTIAL FOR INJURY. For instance, the time I dropped an eighty-five-pound bar on myself during a clean-and-jerk. It hit my chin, bounced off my clavicle, and rolled down my legs. The bruises from that one were not only very awkward to explain but lasted for weeks. One other thing to note: They still use some older lifts that have since been discarded as too injury-inducing by most lifters. Several of their favorites regularly come up on all of the "Top Ten Lifts to Avoid" lists.

5. IT USED MY COMPETITIVENESS AGAINST ME. This was both a pro and a con. It inspired me to do more, but there were a few times Gym Buddy Allison and I nearly killed ourselves trying to "keep up" with those mythical half-man/half-beasts on the CrossFit boards.

This is one serious workout. I loved it. I hated it. I loved to hate it. I now know that I can bang out a half dozen pull-ups—which I definitely couldn't do before. I can also now say that I have dropped some very heavy weights on myself and lived to tell the tale. Plus, I have never in my life got so many compliments on my arms.

When people ask me what the best workout for achieving the most results in the shortest amount of time is, I tell them CrossFit. While there are several good reasons why it might not be a good idea for certain people, I have never come across a workout as effective for building muscle as this one.

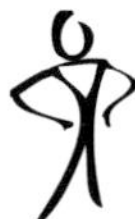

P·E·R·S·O·N·A·L | E·S·S·A·Y

Locker Room Drama

My locker room drama started and ended with the showers. Sixth grade P.E. ("Phy Ed" if you're from Minnesota) found me at the end of a long line of body-conscious girls wrapped in thin towels, each waiting her turn to wash off the sweat from dodge ball. Despite the fact that huddling against a wall staring at boys didn't really work up a sweat and, more importantly, that everyone would see you naked, showering wasn't optional, and our gym teacher stood by the door with a clipboard making sure no one skipped out on their hygienic duty. As I waited my turn, I watched the girl in front of me. She walked up to the shower, flashed her towel open in a quick five-second burst and then quickly stepped away, blushing and unwashed. But she got her name checked off the list and nobody saw if she had pubic hair yet, so I did the same. Plus her bangs, fluffed and aqua-netted a la Debbie Gibson (first tape I ever owned!), survived unscathed. That was important to me since my bangs, combined with my big plastic glasses, were my protection. When the cool kids decided to hawk loogies on me—the same cool kids, by the way, who now friend me on Facebook, causing me to mourn the fact that while you can "poke" someone and give them a "noogie," there is no app for hawking booger juice—my bangs and glasses provided a geek force field that kept the sticky wetness off my actual skin.

Fast forward many years through high school, gymnastics, community theater, dance, and many other opportunities to drop my towel—but I never did. I was the master of clutching my towel with one hand and wriggling out of a wet swimsuit with the other. Then I had children—five of them—and my body was not my own anymore. I became self-conscious in a whole new way, with stretch marks and saggy breasts. In addition, I choose to wear underwear specific to my LDS faith. Like many Muslims and Jews, we wear certain items of clothing that symbolize our commitments to God. They have the added benefit of making us stand out in a crowded locker room. Afraid of questioning or disapproving stares, I moved into the bathroom stalls to change, thereby introducing a whole new degree of difficulty called Don't Drop Your Cell Phone In the Toilet.

And then one day, there I was wrapped in an itty-bitty gym-issue towel, lined up at the shower stalls again. At our YMCA there are only three stalls but a whole wall of open showers, and yet all of us women—old, young, mothers, teens—waited for the private booths. I was running late and had to pick up my son from preschool. Those of you with children will understand that there is nothing more harrowing than missing your child's bus or pickup. Not only does the abandoned child commence hysterical crying exactly two seconds after his comrades-in-paint-smocks have left, but I swear the teachers, irritated by lateness, add to the horror by saying things like, "Well, if your mom doesn't come soon the janitor will just have to put you in the toy closet for the evening, ha ha!" Never incur the wrath of a preschool teacher is all I'm saying.

After a few anxious minutes of watch checking and toe tapping, I decided that this was it. I was done with the towel. I stepped out of line, hung it on a peg and turned on the shower.

Making a quick decision to face the wall and showcase my cellulite rather than advertise my inattentiveness to bikini-line maintenance, I didn't see what the line was doing. But a few seconds later the shower next to me turned on. I looked over to see a woman with whom I'd just done TurboKick. Catching my eye, she laughed and blushed and mumbled about how silly it all was—"It's not like I have anything you all haven't seen!"—and we got clean. Soon another shower turned on. And then another. I glanced around at all of the saggy and smooshy, the Mormon and the atheist, the taut and the wrinkled, the pregnant and the post-partum. And you know who cared? Nobody.

After that, the locker room dynamic changed considerably for me. I no longer agonized about changing in a stall. (Although Gym Buddy Allison chooses to do so, which led to an interesting conversation shouted over toilets the other day when she discovered a need to borrow a sports bra, and I wasn't sure which stall she was in and proceeded to pelt random strangers with it until I found her.) And while I don't roam around starkers having deep conversations with strangers and blow-drying my pits, I no longer care if people see me tucking my mummy tummy skin into my pants or if they think my underwear is funny or even if they notice my strange predilection to matching my cute socks to my cute bras. Because we're all more alike than we are different.

And, also, now I never have to wait for a shower.

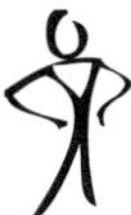

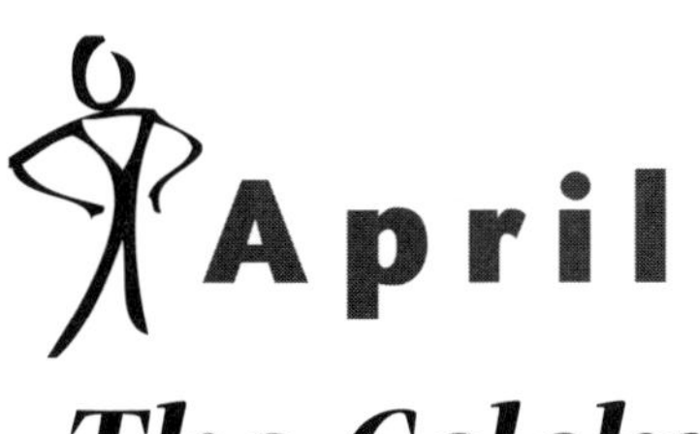

chapter four

April
The Celebrity Workout

Given the amount of press celebrities get (and, to a lesser extent, their trainers), it was inevitable I would have to try a workout designed for, by, and pimped out by people with better hair, better teeth, and better bodies than mine. What I didn't realize was that I would end up acting like a celebrity. And not in a good way.

The Theory

If you've been breathing for the better part of two decades, you've heard of Gwyneth Paltrow and a little somebody I like to call Madonna. (Yes, *that* Madonna so no genuflecting necessary; although, I daresay working out with her would be a religious experience.) Despite their differing physiques—tall, willowy, and blond for the former, and short, muscular, and blond for the latter—they both use the same personal trainer, a woman who has taken on c-list celeb status all on her own for everything but her workouts. Meet Tracy Anderson, a short, willowy blond (noticing a trend?) and the inventor of the creatively named Tracy Anderson Method.

The main selling point of her workout is that if you want to look like a dancer, you need to act like a dancer. This does make sense; to a certain extent, you are what you do. Think swimmers with their powerful shoulders, gymnasts with their muscular thighs, and pro wrestlers with their hair extensions. And basketball players and their long limbs! Oh, wait, that would be genetics. Of course the question then becomes does the sport shape the athlete or do athletes with that shape gravitate towards that particular sport? To wit, will working out like a ballerina give me the classical lithe, lean shape of one?

This promise particularly intrigued Gym Buddy Allison because as the one of us who puts on muscle the easiest and has the lowest body fat percentage, she said CrossFit bulked her thighs out. Girlfriend loves her muscle, but she also loves her current jeans. While it is a myth that women can bulk out like men—we simply don't have the testosterone for that kind of look—it is certainly true that a girl can become more muscular-looking than she prefers. This societal double standard of wanting women to be long, lean, and "toned" but not muscular would become a recurring theme over the course of the year of Great Fitness Experiments, as we discovered the different ways each Gym Buddy's unique body type responded to the different exercises.

The underlying principle to the Method—not that she ever comes right out and says this (do they ever?)—is lots of medium-intensity cardio combined with a low-weight, high-rep weight lifting plan. Celebrities that work out with Anderson personally (at her $900-a-month gym in Manhattan or L.A.) will also get thrice weekly workouts on a Pilates Reformer machine that she modified. For all of this, she promises you will look like Britney pre-mental breakdown.

The Workout

THE TRACY ANDERSON METHOD IS BASED ON doing three key fitness activities every week: the dance cardio, the strength portion, and the custom Reformer. Not being celebrities, the Gym Buddies and I had to get creative to do this workout. In addition to not looking like celebrities, we also don't have the resources of celebrities, so rather than buy Tracy Anderson's pricey program, I cobbled one together based on the multitude of press interviews she did and her own promo material on her Web site. (I know, this ought to have been called The Great Cheapskate Experiment.)

Dance Cardio

Anderson recommends thirty minutes several days a week of some form of dance cardio. Don't like to dance? Then she recommends a running/skipping/galloping combo that has the double bonus of toning your quads while simultaneously providing free entertainment to anyone watching you. The cardio piece was the easiest part of the Anderson Method to implement, as it turns out the Gym Buddies already love to dance. (The Grand Canyon is overrated; if you see one thing before you die, it's gotta be Gym Buddy Megan's "tootsie roll.") And me? Well, if you've had the pleasure of seeing me in public, you know if there is music—even Musak, much to my children's chagrin—then I will be dancing. Grocery stores, parking lots, church dinners, you play it and I will swing it. So Monday nights we Hip Hopped, Wednesdays we Zumba'ed (an aerobicized form of Latin dancing), and Fridays and Saturdays Turbo Jennie whipped our butts in TurboKick (with moves like "the stripper squat" and the "Beyonce bounce" in between kicks and punches, it's definitely very dancey).

Strength

Think low weight and high reps, '80s style (I'll leave the thong leotard and Aqua Net bangs to your discretion.) The theory behind light weight/high reps is that it builds "longer, leaner, more compact muscle." Since Anderson recommends to "never lift anything over three pounds; it will make you bulk out"—she is not, apparently, a mother nor a Costco shopper—we were in luck, as our YMCA has a bountiful supply of candy-colored teeny dumbbells. Unintended bonus: We now had the option of matching our weights to our outfits! Somehow I think Gwyneth would approve.

In addition to "toning," Anderson says to focus only on the smaller, supporting muscles. Avoid training your large muscles at all costs. Says Tracy, "Don't go the gym and do tons of leg presses. Better to stay home and do one hundred plies or something that's not going to bulk you up." Not wanting to mess up this most critical portion of the program and also having no experience as a ballerina, I took a workout that Anderson gave to the *Daily Mail* newspaper and combined it with the Lotte Berk Method developed by an actual ballerina.

This is what the Gym Buddies and I did three days a week:

100 V-arm raises with 3-pound dumbbells

100 shoulder pulses with 3-pound dumbbells, each arm

100 bicep curls with 3-pound dumbbells, each arm

100 tricep kickbacks with 3- pound dumbbells, each arm

50 first position plie squats

50 second position plie squats

5 sets of diamond squats, holding for 10 seconds and alternated with 10 pelvic tilts

25 sideways squats with inner thigh squeeze

25 sideways squats with pelvic tilts

30 standing arabesque pulses, each leg

30 seated pretzel lifts, each leg

30 leg lifts from plank position, each leg

100 V-up sit-ups

100 yoga crunches

100 regular crunches

The Lotte Berk Method recommends that you stretch each muscle group immediately after working it to "elongate the muscle you just contracted." I don't know if there is any scientific basis for that but it sure feels good, so the Gym Buddies and I threw in a few stretches—raising our arms and such to make them as ballerina-like as possible—after each muscle.

The Modified Pilates Reformer

Not only do we not have access to a regular Pilates Reformer—a cross between a medieval torture device and a rowing machine, if you've never seen one—but the Gym Buddies and I certainly do not have access to an Anderson-customized Reformer. In all the interviews she gave, Anderson credits up to two hours a day on her Reformer as one of the keys to her clients' success. However, in the program she sells to the plebian masses on her Web site, it is not used. So I compromised by using my extensive fitness connections to swing us a few free traditional Reformer lessons (read: The Y was offering a free intro to Pilates to all its members).

In the Gym

AFTER DOING CROSSFIT LAST MONTH, the dancer workout was a huge change for us. The first thing to feel the hurt: our egos. Having spent all of March impressing (or scaring, whatever) all the men on the weight floor with our pull-ups, one-rep-maxes, and Olympic lifts, to go immediately to tossing around three-pounders was a bit of a blow. Of course, we didn't help our case by chatting loudly, giggling, and snapping our gum to help pass the time—the above workout ended up taking us a good hour to seventy-five minutes to complete—like silly pre-teens. The only thing we were lacking was our Miley Cyrus tank tops.

And yet. Other things hurt too. Like actual muscle things. This might surprise you—it sure surprised me—but one hundred reps of anything really, really burns. You thought the stares from lifting three-pound pink weights were bad; you should have seen the stares we got when we were shaking and red-faced lifting three-pound pink weights. We were beginning to respect The Method.

Tricep kickbacks and shoulder raises were old hat for us, but the ballet moves were uncharted territory and it showed. As is often the case, just when I look inept enough to actually hurt myself, a professional steps in. This time it was in the form of a tall, willowy blond (yes, seriously) former ballerina named Julie. After watching us mangle the basic plié by sticking our butts and chests out whilst gripping a handrail (our barre, thank you very much) for dear life, she took us in hand and taught us the basic barre work. It's amazing how much your butt and quads can hurt when you do the move the right way.

Another interesting thing developed during this Experiment. For the first time we acquired a male Gym Buddy. While we have had various men stop in to try different workouts with us, this was the first workout that a man was interested in doing for the entire duration. I'm not sure how to explain this except that he's not gay, and there is a lot of hip thrusting involved in the Lotte Berk

Method. Or perhaps he just enjoyed all the witty banter. Either way, we now had a consistent male opinion!

Out of the Gym

IT WAS INEVITABLE: With things going so well inside the gym, something had to fall apart outside of it. In this case it was a fierce resurgence of my long-battled eating disorder. That's the funny thing about eating disorders—they are pernicious. As soon as I think I have it licked, it mutates into another form and surprises me all over again.

My battle with the scale is one of my earliest memories. I remember dieting and feeling fat at eight years old. At ten I wrote in my journal a detailed exercise plan I had to complete before bed every night. Then, thanks to an overzealous and slightly insensitive middle school health teacher ("Did you really eat all that for lunch, Charlotte?! You should pay more attention to what you're eating!"), I started food journaling and restricting at age twelve. It was a disordered habit I would keep up almost non-stop for the next *eighteen* years. Naturally, the boys in my health class had carte blanche to eat whatever they "needed" to keep up their strength for sports and because they were still growing. Never mind that many of us girls were also in sports and also, duh, still growing.

In high school and college, I flirted with outright anorexia (as did far too many of my friends), always managing to keep my weight just on the safe side of things. Always able to pull back when I really needed to. I never cognizantly thought of the times where I would subsist on a single "fun size" package of candy for an entire day, several days in a row, as restricting. I just thought it was what girls did to stay thin.

Lots of girls I knew did it or things similar to it. Other waitresses at the restaurant I worked at taught me which foods had the least calories and tricks to make all the decadent food we were surrounded by look unappealing so we wouldn't be tempted to eat it. Our dinner breaks turned into competitions to see who could eat the smallest amount of actual food. Girls in my gymnastics classes taught me about not eating before a competition (the lower your weight, the higher you fly!) and then using massive doses of caffeine pills to mask the hunger and keep your energy up. Roommates taught me about "saving calories" by restricting all week so you could eat on a date, and the guy would think you are one of the cool girls who is thin but can eat whatever she wants.

This type of behavior also runs in my family—my grandmother, whom I still adore and think about almost daily despite her being dead for twenty years, was an active bulimic all her adult life. Two cousins were bulimic. Another did several stints in eating disorder clinics. And then of course there was the media—thin movie stars, even thinner fashion models. Even my "health" teacher encouraged disordered eating. I was surrounded, almost from birth, by our culture of thin. Every girl I knew was tainted by it.

And yet my bouts of bad eating were interspersed with longer ones of health because my body's will to survive and thrive was stronger than my willpower to starve. That is, until I met the Very Bad Boyfriend in college. He was my partner on a swing-dance team. He was an amazing dancer and, simultaneously, a sociopath. I saw something good in him and he, likewise, saw something in me: vulnerability. We began to date. The entire time we went out (if you can call it that), he abused me in every way possible. It started out small with little comments about how I was harder to lift than some of the other girls on our team—natural waifs, every last one of them. Then it progressed to screaming vitriol, that I cannot even now bring myself to repeat.

To cope, I did what came naturally—I stopped eating. I pulled out all the tricks I'd ever been taught over the years and combined them with hours of intensely athletic dancing. It worked. VBB complimented me on my protruding hipbones. He liked that his hands could almost span my waist. He was happy. I was nearly destroyed. I fainted after a dance performance. I suffered heart palpitations, dizzy spells, nausea, and insomnia. He finished the job by sexually assaulting me. That was the end of my relationship with him, thanks to good friends and family, but the beginning of a kind of self-loathing I had never experienced before.

After VBB, my weight went up a bit and stabilized. I met a great man who cared about my mind and my soul and honestly thought I was beautiful regardless of a few pounds up or down. I married him, and for a few short years, managed to not think about food or weight at all. The hole in me wasn't gone, but at least it was covered up.

That came to an end when VBB popped back into my life in the most horrific way possible. At the time, I had assumed that I was the only girl he had abused. Turns out he was a serial molester and had only gotten worse during the intervening years. I was contacted by the police and decided to press charges.

My only experience with our legal system being *Law & Order* reruns, I was wholly unprepared for the physical and mental nightmare of a sexual assault case. I was also pregnant with my third child. The interstate court case dragged on nine long months, exactly the length of my pregnancy. The longer it went on, the more I deteriorated. I couldn't eat. I couldn't sleep. Despite being pregnant, I quickly reached the lowest weight I'd ever been. I thought about suicide every single day. The baby inside me was the only thing that stopped me from actually doing it. VBB finally plea-bargained and got a year in prison, with time served. The very next day, my son was born. Hale and hearty at ten pounds, he was a beautiful child. His mother was broken.

With the court case ended, everyone assumed I would feel empowered and vindicated and quickly ease back into my old, perfect life as wife, teacher, and mother. I think they assumed that because that is what they so desperately wanted for me. What did I want for me? I wanted desperately to finally heal. I thought being healthy physically would help me mentally. But this time my disordered eating snuck up on me as my quest for ultimate health devolved into orthorexia, a newly coined term for people who restrict their food based on health reasons as opposed to wanting to be thin. In fact, I'm told it's the new "in" eating disorder in the Hollywood set. Yay, me.

I saw a therapist who was pretty good at helping me work through my damage from the abusive relationship. But when it came to my disordered eating, she was worse than unhelpful.

She wanted tips. Every week as I shrank before her very eyes, she would ask in awe how I did it. Somewhat overweight herself, she pressed until I actually gave her a how-to, which she then promised to implement. At last we both realized that she had problems with her own self image and that our relationship had moved far from being therapeutic. So I stopped seeing her. But I still hurt. I just covered it up better.

And then in March, during the CrossFit Experiment, *20/20* came calling. The venerable ABC news program had found an article I had written about my orthorexia and wanted to do a show on the eating disorder. I, thinking it would be a great way to get the message out about this new insidious illness and save others from my fate, readily agreed. The thing that I hadn't considered about being on TV is that everyone is going to be, you know, watching you. For a girl with so many pre-existing body-image issues, it was a nightmare. For the first time, I began to understand why so many celebrities have disordered eating patterns.

As we prepped for the six-hour taped interview (John Stossel was doing the piece! Not that I got to meet him. In fact the producer waved his hand vaguely left of camera and instructed me to "talk to the hand.") with endless e-mails and phone calls, it became apparent: Talking about eating disorders was giving me one.

After the initial phone call from the *20/20* producer, the panic quickly set in. Me on national television? My house on national television? My husband and I were in the middle of a large-ish remodeling project on our Totally Rad 80s House, and it was in no condition to be seen, much less filmed. We could either try to temporarily cover everything up, or we could push through and finish the renovation in a hurry.

Being the neurotic perfectionist that I am, I opted for the latter. Oh, and did I mention that my dear husband was out of town on a business trip until just two days before the interview? And that I had three tiny, sticky-fingered children that love to "help"? Just in the nick of time, I was saved by my wonderful friends, Gym Buddies Allison and Candice, as well as Personal Trainer DarLee who showed up with paint rollers and nail guns and stayed until the wee hours of the morning, several nights in a row. We finished painting and cleaning mere hours before the camera crew showed up. It was intense.

So I wasn't sleeping. And I'm one of those people who when they are stressed out, can't eat. But I was still hitting all of my workouts because that's how I release stress. The end result? In the month between the phone call and the interview, I lost so much weight that I went from a "healthy" BMI of 19 to "officially underweight" according to the World Health Organization.

I did realize what was happening but gave myself permission to let my body do its thing because I was so stressed out. This has happened before, and I'd always quickly gained the weight back as soon as the stress passes. But this time there was a difference. As I lost the weight, everyone began complimenting me. And I mean everyone. Only two people said anything remotely negative. One was my mother, who commented, "Wow, your collar bone is really prominent. I don't think I've ever seen it stick out so much." The other was Gym Buddy Allison, who took me aside one day at the gym to ask, "Exactly how much more weight are you planning on losing? I think you should stop."

I don't think I am the vainest girl around—I'll easily go days without make-up. I don't care if people see me sweat. I know I have plenty of physical flaws—but I'm not immune to compliments, and so I kept up the not eating. People at church stopped me to tell me how fantastic I looked. It might have been my imagination, but I swear I was getting better service at stores. People at the gym began gushing over my new figure and asking me how I did it. One woman even told me I had "the perfect figure." I had a BMI of 17, hadn't menstruated in months, and could count all my ribs. In my chest. Perfect, indeed.

I was too embarrassed to tell anyone what had happened. Here I was on television (the *20/20* segment didn't air until September 2008, but in the interim I also appeared on Fox's morning show to discuss the perils of anorexia) talking about overcoming eating disorders, and I still had one! And so I didn't mention it to the Gym Buddies. I didn't tell my family. I didn't even write about it on my blog, where I'm notorious for being a chronic over-sharer.

All of that silence worked to my detriment. I began to panic. I wanted to stay underweight. And yet the only way to do that was to continue on my unhealthy cycle of self-destruction. The moment of truth finally came when *20/20* called in September, at the last minute, looking for one more picture of me "at my thinnest." I guess all the ones I had sent them before weren't shocking enough in a media age where "eating disorder" is typically illustrated with a picture of a sixty-pound shell of a human being—even though the ill effects of undereating begin long before that. At last, frustrated over the chronic phone calls and e-mails demanding more sick pictures, I sent them one I'd been holding back. It was the one they ended up using in the commercials, on their Web site, and of course in the show. And it was one taken of me that day, in September.

While I loved all the compliments, the effects of maintaining such a low weight were beginning to wear on me. My stamina in my workouts was affected as I tired much faster, got sore more easily and stayed sore longer. In classic anorexic fashion, my heart rate became erratic, my sleep was disturbed, I hadn't had a period in months, and I was cold all the time. I hate being cold. I hate being tired. I hate being hungry. And I hate that the world I live in is so messed up that everyone thinks I'm beautiful only when I'm cold, tired, and hungry.

At the end of the *20/20* interview, the producer asked me to "sum it all up." What would I say to someone who is currently struggling with orthorexia? I answered, "Know that those who love you will still love you—even if you aren't perfect." Oh, the irony.

The Results

IF MY MINOR BRUSH WITH CELEBRITY CAUSED me to crash and burn so much, I can only imagine what real celebrities must go through with the constant media scrutiny. Perhaps it was this newfound sympathy for the rich and famous that helped me take my "Celebrity Workout" more seriously, or perhaps it was the fact that, despite all the pastel rubber 'bells, it actually gave a good burn, but I saw results.

After I overcame my initial dubiousness, there were many things I liked about the workout. First of all, it was hard. You think three-pounders are wimpy? Do 100 reps. You will want to gnaw your own arm off just to escape the pain. I will never ever make fun of someone for using the baby weights again. Secondly, you could bounce quarters off my perky butt (but if you do, be warned that I'm keeping the quarters—all that therapy doesn't pay for itself!). Quite honestly, I don't know if I have ever done glute-ham exercises as effective as the ballerina moves. That pretzel move left us feeling like we had a nail stuck in each butt cheek afterward. Third, you can call me Gumby—all that stretching made it possible for me to do all my splits again. Lastly, I swear my waist was smaller, and I had visible definition in my top two abs. (No word yet from the remaining four, but an expedition has been sent out. They've got to be there somewhere.) Seriously, though, 300 sit-ups a day!

Unfortunately, you have to take into account that I contaminated my own results with my budding eating disorder. Were the visible abs compliments of all those sit-ups—like I'd like to believe—or simply from losing so much weight? Thankfully, I have the results from the other Gym Buddies. Allison, the one concerned with her "bulky" thighs (that were not big at all—I'm not the only one in the gym with issues), saw results by losing up to three-quarters of an inch each off her waist, thighs, arms and calves. Megan and Candice, while they didn't see any changes in

Best Moment

In a world of matchy-matchy Nike outfits, workout clothing can sometimes get a little boring for a girl whose sartorial taste can best be described as "quirky." Thankfully, I discovered a Web site (URL redacted to protect their good name—I can't hold them responsible for what happened next) that detailed 101 ways to cut up a T-shirt. Brilliant! So I took a lime-green striped Walmart T-shirt, and with a few artful cuts had turned it into a halter top reminiscent of a 1940s swimsuit, complete with little bows on the straps! It looked adorable . . . until I began to sweat and the 100 percent cotton started to stretch. If before T-shirt surgery, the shirt had merely made my boobs look like they were in prison, ten minutes into my workout, the convicts were definitely escaping. And just like in the movies, the girls were trying to dig a tunnel to freedom. It's bad enough that this workout had enough hip thrusting in it to make hula girls blush, but now I was going to have to add stripper to my resume. By the end of the workout, my top was literally in tatters. I was Cinderella in a sports bra but without the magical singing mice. Thank heavens for Nike after all.

inches, did feel like their clothes fit a bit better. And for the lone man in our Experiment? He credits all those plies and arabesques with increasing his muscle endurance—and his tolerance for talk about sports bras, birth control, and hair removal (we kindly left off childbirth, he is still single after all).

The main downside to this type of high-volume workout is the boredom. How many times can you count to 100 before silliness takes over? It also took forever to complete. If you like your gym experiences closer to In-N-Out Burger than a Japanese steakhouse, this workout—easily two hours a day if you add in the Reformer or dance cardio—will drive you nuts. Third, it's embarrassing. I know, I'm the girl who cherry drops from the pull-up bar and handstand walks on the weight floor, but there was just something particularly agonizing about those teeny tiny little dumbbells. My pride did suffer. The most significant downside was that it doesn't hit every body part. Our chests, backs, and lats became so neglected that we started adding in those exercises on our "off" days because we were afraid of losing muscle there.

Our verdict? It's definitely worth throwing this workout into the mix a few times a month but any more than that, and you'll know why Madonna always has that wild look in her eye.

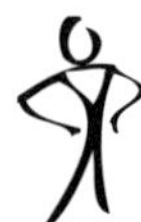

P·E·R·S·O·N·A·L | ·E·S·S·A·Y

Body Insecurity Is Contagious

I didn't know there was a problem with my nose until I was twenty-four. Really and truly. I walked around this planet for twenty-four years wearing that thing in front of my face, and I never once noticed anything awry in the mirror. But I learned better that fateful spring morning.

A new mom, I had taken my nine-month-old to the park to "play" (Who was I kidding? The kid was a veritable potted plant, except I had to keep turning him away from the sun instead of towards it. Didn't want him to get sunburned, you see. In Seattle. In March. Like I said, new mom.) when a stranger struck up a conversation with me. She was also a mom of a little boy, who was enthusiastically ignoring all the cool playground equipment and eating the woodchips instead, and she lived in my neighborhood.

As our conversation progressed, she declared to me, in a way that strangers only do with other strangers, that she was actually at the park because she was going in for plastic surgery that afternoon. Usually she worked, but had taken a "vacation" to get "it" fixed. And "these" she whispered despite us being the only ones in the whole park, gesticulating at her smallish chest. "That's for my husband."

"Ever since I was fourteen, I've been saving money to get my nose done," she explained. "And now I'm twenty-eight. It's about time!" I nodded sympathetically as I squinted at her nose. It looked . . . just like my nose.

"What are they going to fix?" I asked, hoping she would say a deviated septum or something.

"OMG! THIS!" She stuck her face in my face. A bump on the bridge of her nose came into focus.

"Oh, okay," I mumbled. The damage was done. As soon as I got in the car, I checked my nose in the rear view mirror. Bump? Yep. (Go ahead, flip to the cover and check out my nose. It's there in all its un-Photoshopped glory!) When I walked in my house, I dropped wee Potted Plant on the floor in front of some toys and ran to my big mirror to examine my schnoz from every angle.

Where did that bump come from? Surely as a child I had that little button nose that children are, well, famous for. I broke my nose falling off a hammock in sixth grade—was that when it happened? How had I never noticed it before? Was that why Jake broke up with me my freshman year of college? I mean all he said was, "This doesn't feel right." But maybe he meant: "Your nose is hideous! I can't pass that genetic freak show on to my kids!"

My kids! I ran out to look at Potted Plant. He had a tiny perfect ski-jump nose—Gerber-baby cute if not for the perpetual stream of snot that oozed from it. I sighed with relief but made a mental note to be on the lookout for it as he grew up. Although, I rationalized, he was a boy, and the world is more forgiving of mogul-ed noses on men.

After that, I had to check my profile in every reflective surface that came my way. I'm sure people thought I was the vainest woman they'd ever seen. Vain I was not. Terrified is what I was. My husband assured me that he loved me in spite of it, which only led me to realize that he'd seen my bump all along and never told me about it!

The Playground Lady's voice echoed through my head for weeks.

Until I talked to my friend Gym Buddy Eleanor, pouring out all my trite yet expansive worries on her shoulder. When I finished she laughed her butt off, pointed to her own nose that could best be described as Jewish, and replied "That's why I accessorize with expensive shoes." Her ability to laugh at and even embrace her "flaw" completely changed my perspective.

Why am I telling you this story? Because it is important how we talk about our bodies. Even if it is just to a stranger in the park, but especially if it is in front of our children. We should also take care in talking about other people's bodies. I'm convinced that our extreme criticism of celebrities only eats away at our own self-worth.

Two-and-a-half years ago, I decided to try a little experiment and cut out TV and movies. That's right—all of 'em. Once I got over wondering what was happening on *Grey's Anatomy*, it actually wasn't as bad as I thought it would be. But the biggest change was how I felt about myself. Once I wasn't bombarded with "America's Next Top Model" and "Hollywood's Top 50 Sexiest Women" and even the more subtle super-skinny-and-oh-so-empowered Dr. Meredith Grey, I felt better about who I was. Although I still struggle with liking myself, cutting out TV made a huge difference in helping me think more positively about myself. I didn't even realize how far I'd come until I spoke to an old friend who was punishingly critical of her (beautiful) post-baby body and was able to show her my tiger-claw stretch marks with love and even pride.

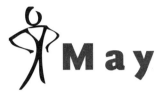

chapter five

May

The Action Hero Workout

WHAT DOES EVERY LITTLE GIRL BORN IN THE '80S want to grow up to be? She-Ra: Princess of Power! (Or possibly Rainbow Brite—those moon boots are rad.) I remember meeting She-Ra when I was in kindergarten. She was at the local suburban mall complete with dance tights, metallic underwear, and Sword of Truth. She made the leather cone bra cool long before Xena ever wore it. And there was I, in my Wonder Woman (Wonder Woman/She-Ra, same diff, right?) Underoos that my mom actually let me wear out of the house. I was awesome and not just because I put Madonna to shame with my underwear-as-outerwear style: I was a superhero.

As I grew older, my fondness for female action stars never waned. There was a brief hiatus in the '90s where I was too concerned with being angsty and, like, watching, like, *My So-Called Life*, to, like, kick any bad-guy butt. (Although my grunge years were not a waste—if SAT grading ever goes out of style, at least I can fall back on my hemp-necklace-making skills.) But then I grew up and got married and had kids who gave me my fill of cartoon inanity, so I moved on to real-life action heroes. It all started when my mother one day—kindly and crazily—compared me to Jennifer Garner, pre-*Alias* cancellation. We both liked to rock climb and kickbox! No matter that she wore pleather minis and go-go boots while she roundhoused and my "wardrobe" consists entirely of shirts that have been puked on, we were like soul sisters.

So it was kismet when I came across Valerie Waters, personal trainer to the stars in general and Jennifer Garner in particular. She had devised a workout specifically to help Jennifer get her butt-kicking body back after having her daughters. If it worked for Jennifer Garner, it would work for me, right?

The Theory

BEING TOO CHEAP TO BUY HER E-BOOK *Red Carpet Ready*, I'm not exactly sure what her methodology is. (True story: I fell in love with my husband when he showed up for our first date with a two-for-one sandwich coupon and a warm two-liter of Coke in his trunk. Nothing says romance like a good BOGO!) Fortunately for me, she has a blog on which she posts sample workouts. Judging from these, her workouts are based around two things: 1) circuits that incorporate both weights and cardio into one workout, and 2) cutely named equipment that she designed, such as the Val-Slides and the Val-Band. The thing I liked right away was she incorporated a lot of exercises that I'd never done before, such sliding push-ups, sliding curtsey lunges, and other movements reminiscent of the Ice Capades. Even better, she provided step-by-step pictures of how to do everything! Cheapskate bliss!

The Workout

NOT BEING SURE HOW MANY DAYS A WEEK to do her Val-Circuits nor how much or what kind of cardio to do in between—all stuff I'd know if I'd bought the book—I did what I usually do when I don't know something. I make it up. So I devised a program where we did two circuits from the Val-Blog (I didn't make that up, that's what it is really called), alternating them on Monday, Wednesday, and Friday. Each circuit is repeated three times to complete the workout. On Tuesday, Thursday, and Saturday, we did our normal cardio-lovin' routine.

In the Gym

Pop Quiz!

Q: "So what's up with the paper plates?"

a. Redecorating. Don't you think our little Dixie plates with the orange flowers add a nice punch of color to the Y?

b. Why should the kids have all the crafty fun? We're making sheep puppets today! We got the cotton balls from the first-aid box.

c. Having an imaginary picnic. It's our new "air" diet. We're losing weight like crazy. They warned us, though, that hallucinations are a possible side effect. Good thing that's not happening—right, Batman?

d. I'm too cheap to buy a Val-Slide, but I still wanna be an Action Hero(ine).

(See page 100 for quiz answer!)

The first item of importance was to determine our "inner superhero" via a super-reliable Internet quiz. (What, now you're too good for Facebook quizzes?) I'm The Flash. No, I'm not one overcoat and a subway shy of a police escort. It means that, according to the Superhero Quiz, I'm "fast, flirtatious, and virtuous"—aka The Flash. I only have two problems with this: 1) Can one be both fast, flirtatious, *and* virtuous? They kinda seem to rule each other out. 2) I am not a man. But whatevs, once the Gym Buddies and I all had our Superhero IDs firmly in place, we moved into the gym.

The second item of importance was to acquire the necessary equipment. See, I'm cheap. I might have mentioned that. Some of you might think that not having the proper equipment would compromise the integrity of our Experiment. I choose to think it enhances it, as lots of people—most people, really—won't have access to specialized equipment. But should that hold anyone back from being able to do a Sea Witch Crawl? Never!

Upon close examination of the Val-Slides, we decided they were two pieces of plastic that one could use to move across carpet—you know, like those carpet skates they make for kids. The circuits called for the use of the Val-Slides in almost every exercise, placed either under the feet or the hands, so we had to come up with something. Over the course of the month, we tried many substitutes for the Val-Slides. This had the dual effect of working our muscles and making us the laughing stock of the gym. I swear people started lining up early just to see what else we would drag in from home and then try to slide on.

Our first attempt was using dishrags on the wood floor of the basketball gym. The ballers loved us. Really they did. Yeah we got hit with a lot of stray basketballs, but I'm sure those were just accidents. (Unlike the time an old man deliberately hawked a loogie over the railing of the second story track onto to me while I was holding plank on the gym floor below. I will have you know that I did not come out of plank. And, also, my Hepatitis B shots are now up to date.) The dishrags, unfortunately, didn't work very well as they crumpled up underneath our hands, not to mention all the times we got them confused with our sweat towels and mopped our sweaty brows with feet detritus. Although the YMCA janitors bought us a thank-you card, so it was all worth it in the end. I'm telling you—if there is one Gym Person you really want on your side, it's the janitor.

Up next were paper plates (great until they burned through after one use), Styrofoam plates (not as slidey as you'd think and also bad for the environment), and paper towels (we were desperate). Eventually we settled on two things that worked well: plastic picnic plates—as long as we were careful to get the kind without the knobs on the bottom—and, I kid you not, perfume ads from magazines (the thickness of the paper was the key, plus they made us smell like ginger, lilac, and sandalwood with just a hint of cardamom!) Besides, can you think of a better use for *Cosmopolitan*?

Thankfully, the Val-Band, being just a circle of rubber about one foot in diameter, was much easier to fake, as our Y has a big bucket of random gym equipment including a bunch of bands.

Once equipped, we set off on our circuits. Cutesy names and equipment aside, they were *hard*. They definitely gave us a good burn. We were sore the entire first week. Now that I've got you intrigued, do you want to get in on this slidey action?

The sideways slidey lunge. This is the most elementary of all slidey moves, so start here. Plant one foot on terra firma, put the other one on your Val-Slide/plastic picnic plate/Beyonce "Fierce" Parfum ad. Squatting down into your not-moving leg, slide your other leg out to the side as far as you can. Now slide it back in towards you as you stand up. Your inner thighs have never burned so good! (Unless you've tried to do a bikini wax on yourself at home. Gluing your legs together will hurt much, much worse. Don't ask me how I know this. Ahem.) Be sure to switch sides. Nobody wants uneven butt cheeks.

The slidey push-up. On your toes (you are She-Ra, right?), in perfect push-up position, place one hand on the ground and your other hand on your slide. As you lower yourself down towards the floor, slide your hand out to the side. As you push back up, slide hand in. If you are really awesome, put a slide under *each* hand, moving both hands out and in at the same time. Warning: You will eat it the first time. That's a promise. After you've picked the carpet fibers out of your teeth, get up and try again, but this time from your knees. At least you won't have as far to fall that way!

The slidey worm. Not only will this one work your shoulders, back, arms, and core, but it will also make you the freak show of your gym. Unless you work out at home, and then your cat will just stare at you funny. Anyhow. Start in a "down dog" position (hands and feet on the ground, butt sticking up in the air) with the slide under your feet. Walk your hands out in front of you until you are in a plank position. Now draw in with your abs and pull your feet towards your hands until you are back to the original position. Repeat until you have made it all the way across the floor or until you run into someone.

Out of the Gym

IT STARTED WITH MY DOUBLE CARDIO EXPERIMENT in February, worsened through March, and was exacerbated by two of my television appearances in April. It was inevitable really: May continued the resurgence of my eating disorder. Gym Buddy Allison, who is almost as obsessed with numbers as I am, and I became fixated on our body fat percentage. As I measure it before and after every Experiment, you may wonder what the big deal is about this number. The answer is that besides my obsession with all things numerical, it is one of the better ways to assess your level of health.

A lot of people focus on weight, but the problem is that muscle is more dense than fat so a "skinny fat" person would appear to be more healthy than a very muscular person. This is the primary downfall of the BMI, one of the many reasons it is not a good indicator of health. In addition, the number on the scale is affected by a myriad of factors, such as the time of the month (for women), how much salt you've eaten recently, and how irritating your significant other is being. (Side note: Please never ever say, "A pound of muscle weighs more than a pound of fat." They are both a pound, thereby making them equivalent. I know what you mean when you say that, but it still bugs me. And since I know you all live with the express purpose of not irritating me, I thank you.)

It is generally accepted that looking at the percentage of your body weight made up of fat is a more meaningful number than just scale weight. Of course, if you want a picture of your overall health, body fat percentage is just one of many important numbers.

How To Measure Your Body Fat

If you watch *The Biggest Loser* or *Dr. Phil* (Dr. Phil on *The Biggest Loser*? A product-placement gold mine!), then you are probably familiar with the Tanita scale. Scales that measure body fat percentage, also known as bioelectrical impedance scales, range from the cheap, low-tech variety (which I have) to the crazy-tricked-out-make-your-low-riding-neighbors-rims-jealous variety. You stand on a specially equipped scale, and it sends a small electrical impulse through your body. Depending on how fast it zips back, it calculates your percentage of body fat, as fat and muscle conduct electricity at different rates. Unfortunately water—which our bodies have much of—interferes with the accuracy of this test, making it useless almost to the point of ridiculousness. Despite the hoopla, this is the least accurate way to measure your body fat.

The next best way to get your number is by doing the "pinch test," also known as every eighth grader's gym nightmare. The person—hopefully someone trained in this—grabs chunks of your skin on various parts of your body and measures how thick they are with a metal device called calipers. They add up the numbers, and then, using a chart, tell you your body fat percentage. The first problem with this test is the high rate of user error— read: The more aggressive the trainer, the more skin they grab, and so if you've got Hannibal doing your test, you are going to read "fatter" than you really are. The other problem is that this is not friendly to people who have just had babies or otherwise have handfuls of loose skin just hanging around their bodies. Still, it's better than the body fat scales for accuracy, especially if you have the same person measure you every time (just make sure your trainer is not a sadist).

But the best way to check your fat is either with a Bod Pod (not widely available, plus it takes forty-five minutes, is crazy expensive, and is not for claustrophobics) or hydrostatic weighing. Allison and I, being who we are, chose the latter option.

Which is how we found ourselves at o-dark-thirty on Saturday morning in a cold, dark pool, being watched by a cadaverous professor and clinging to a metal chair suspended from a crane-like arm in the water. Sound fun yet? After donning my new cherry-red retro suit (so cute!), I jumped in the water, perched on the chair and proceeded to submerge, exhaling every last bit of air from my lungs and then trying to hold myself perfectly still in a modified crunch while I watched black spots dance on my eyelids. Have I ever mentioned that my worst fear is to get stuck in a cave underwater? You wouldn't think that unless you are a scuba diver that this would be a fear you would have to confront in your daily life. Okay, so a 40s-era college pool isn't exactly a cave, and I only had to be underwater for about five seconds at a time, but still that was five seconds of I-can't-breathe panic! Plus, every time I surfaced, I got to hear Gym Buddy Allison laughing at me.

It was all worth it though. Hydrostatic weighing is the gold standard in body fat testing—the only way to get a more accurate reading is to get cut open on the autopsy table. Hydrostatic weighing simply means getting weighed underwater. It works this way: Fat is buoyant, so it makes you float; while lean tissue (muscle, skeleton, and water) are dense so they make you sink. Air also makes you float, which is why you have to get every last bit that you can out of your lungs. So, the more you weigh under water, the less body fat you have. It's the only time in my life when I was actually hoping to put up big numbers on the scale.

Once you get over the initial medieval weirdness of the whole contraption, it's kind of entertaining. Which was good since I had to dunk at least ten times. See, you have to exhale *and* hold still, which, due to the aforementioned panic issue, was tough for me. Most people nail the test in four tries or less. I stopped counting after eight, much to Allison's amusement.

What the Numbers Mean

So now you have your number, what do you do with it? According to most charts, the normal range for women is 25–31 percent (18–25 percent for men). Fit chicas check in around 21–24 percent (14–17 percent for men). Athletes are 14–20 percent (6–13 percent for men). Don't forget that your body requires a certain amount of "essential fat" to pad your organs and run your brain which is 10–12 percent for women and 2–4 percent for men.

Generally, lower is better. It means more of your body weight is comprised of lean tissue, and less is made up of fat. But I must point out that, like weight, a "zero" means dead. If you don't know what a woman looks like at a very low body fat percentage, just watch any female body building competition—competitors often drop to a temporary low of 5–10 percent for the competition—to refresh your memory. Plus women need estrogen to maintain their bone density, and estrogen needs fat. Dropping below the essential level can permanently damage your bones, stop your period, and cause malabsorption of vitamins.

So it was a testament to my distorted body image that when I clocked in at an unholy 13 percent, my first thought was, "No way! I still have five pounds of fat I need to lose! I still have a mummy tummy! And check out these thighs!" The professor looked at me with a clinical gleam in his eye and commented only, "I think you are the lowest female I've ever tested. I'm warning you, don't go any lower."

I left his office feeling very disheartened. How could I have no more body fat to lose—literally—and still be able to pinch an inch on my waist? I'd been promised by every fitness professional on the planet that once I got below a certain percentage—most say 16 percent—that not only would I have visible abs, but I'd also have the body of my dreams. I couldn't see my abs and, worse, I still hated the way I looked.

Female Athlete Triad

The rational part of my brain (I haven't completely killed it off yet) kicked in. While some women continue to menstruate at 13 percent body fat, I hadn't had a period since who knows when. I knew from all my reading about the "female athlete triad"—a syndrome characterized by disordered eating, amenorrhea, and osteoporosis—that the consequences for continuing on in this path could be severe. I already had the first two symptoms down pat. I was terribly afraid of the third.

I had started out this journey to get healthy for myself and for my kids, and here I was setting myself up for fragile, brittle bones. How was I supposed to be the active, involved mother and grandmother I had always pictured myself being if I was afraid of breaking a hip at thirty? The truth was starting to break through the madness, but I didn't change my ways until I got a real wake-up call the following month. (Oh yes, the next chapter is a fun one! Breakdowns are involved, both mental and physical!)

June found me in my doctor's office complaining of several months of being chronically cold (it was 70 degrees and I was wearing yoga pants, a long-sleeve T-shirt, a hoodie, and socks), depression, irritability, sudden weight gain, excessive fatigue and muscle soreness, and, worst of all for a writer, a mental "fogginess" that is just not like me. (I want to apologize to all of my friends and family members who had the misfortune of speaking to me during that time as I was perennially pissy.) My doc, after much scanning, prodding, and blood sucking, informed me that my thyroid seemed to be under-functioning.

Hypothyroidism is a fairly common malady, especially in women, and it does run in my family, but I was confused—why would I suddenly have a problem now? I had none of the risk factors for it (over fifty, pregnant, or lactating) and have not had problems with it in the past.

And then she mentioned something interesting—hypothyroidism in younger people is linked to overtraining syndrome. For those of you uninitiated in the die-hard fitness parlance, overtraining syndrome is, according to body building.com, "Training too hard and too long, with insufficient rest, which leads to burnout and decreased performance." There are two types of OT: sympathetic, which mainly affects power athletes like lifters and sprinters; and parasympathetic, which mainly affects endurance athletes.

"But, Charlotte, you are not an athlete!" 'Tis true, but I am dumb enough to train hard like one. Well, like an uneducated one at any rate. The sorry truth is that it is us wannabe athletes that are the most susceptible to this syndrome. Real athletes have coaches and doctors and water boys and ESPN commentators monitoring their every vital sign to nip this kind of thing in the bud. I just had denial.

There is only one cure for overtraining: rest. And lots of it. My instinct when something isn't working for me is to push harder and go farther. My instincts suck. According to most sources, you are supposed to take one week off of exercise for every twelve weeks of intense training. At this point I hadn't taken a week off in years. I'd barely taken a day off since my last baby was born. The longer you have overtrained, the more rest you need. Whitney Myers, an Olympic hopeful that I read about in a *New York Times* profile, ended up so fatigued that she required six months of rest.

After discussing it with my doctor and for the first time 'fessing up to my exercise addiction, she advised me to take two weeks off and then come back in for more blood work. I immediately tried to bargain her down. "How about just one week?" I pleaded. "How about you get therapy?" she replied and wrote down the name and number of an eating disorder clinic.

Not good for a girl in the middle of a Great Fitness Experiment! And yet I knew I had to do it. My hardest "Experiment" of the entire year was coming out to the Gym Buddies and on my blog—everyone was amazingly supportive and encouraging when I finally called a therapist and started out-patient treatment for compulsive over-exercising. I would stay in treatment for the next nine months.

The Results

THE VALERIE WATERS ACTION HERO WORKOUTS were a good burn, but Experimentally speaking weren't a huge change, as we were just swapping out one strength routine for another. I imagine if we'd done her whole *Red Carpet Ready* program—that includes dietary advice in addition to her circuits—we'd probably have seen more of a difference.

What I Liked

1. THE "VAL-SLIDES" (or paper/plastic plates in our case) were a nice change of pace. The moves were novel and interesting. Fun, too!

2. IT WAS A REALLY GOOD BURN. As long as we kept moving quickly through the circuits, our heart rates stayed up most of the time. We were pretty sore too, especially the first week.

3. I REALLY LIKED HOW HER MOVES INCORPORATED BALANCE along with the strength. Plus just about every move made my abs sore!

4. SUZANNE SOMMERS will be glad to know I no longer need her thigh master as this workout rocks the legs and butt!

What I Didn't Like

1. THEY ARE L-O-N-G! One day Allison and I busted through it as fast as we could and finished the whole thing (all nine circuits!) in forty-six minutes. But we were really pushing it and probably lost some form. On average, it took us an hour to an hour and fifteen to complete. We ended up taking it down to two days a week because of how time consuming it got.

2. BORING. I suppose if I had actually bought her book then I would have had more workouts to choose from, but let's just say that Allison and I did a little celebratory dance of joy when we finished. It doesn't help with the monotony that you repeat each circuit three times.

3. IT HITS MOST OF THE MAJOR BODY PARTS, but it was still lacking in a few areas. For example, there was only one shoulder exercise and it only hit the top delt. (Is that actually a body part?

Worst Moment

I have always wanted to run a marathon but the steep entry fees combined with my innate cheapness have always held me back. So one day the brilliant thought occurred to me that I needn't pay anyone for the privilege of running 26.2 miles! I could do it all by myself! Which I did. Not many people would be dumb enough to go out and run for four straight hours on a whim, but the worst is yet to come: Unable to miss a workout, as soon as I finished my run, I rushed home to get ready for my TurboKick class.

My husband met me at the door. As soon as he realized my intent, he put his foot down. "This is too much. You can't go to the gym." Nobody tells me I can't do something. "I'm fine," I retorted. He was unconvinced, and yet he had to leave to go play an Ultimate Frisbee game. In a fit of desperation, he took my car keys and the car with all the car seats in it, so I would be unable to go.

Late and nearly having a panic attack about missing my workout, I waited until he left and then hustled all the kids into his small Honda, seating them in their outgrown car seats that I pulled from the back of the garage. One spare key later, I was on my way to the gym. I hadn't even stopped long enough to eat or drink anything.

I did that hour-long, high-intensity class. By the end I was feeling so nauseous and jelly limbed, I ran out of the class afraid I was going to barf in front of everyone.

My heart started doing funny little flip flops, and for a brief moment, I thought I was going to die. My kids' faces flashed before my eyes, and I experienced horrible regret. Then I fainted.

Fortunately for me, about that time Gym Buddy Paul found me collapsed on the steps and helped me get downstairs where he bought me a Gatorade and waited until I drank it. My first instinct was to decline the sugary drink—I hate drinking my calories—but my pounding heart and clammy hands overruled my neurosis. After twenty minutes of sitting on a couch with my head on my knees, I was finally well enough to get my children and go home. It's the closest to a near-death experience I've ever had, and it was all due to my own stupidity.

I say that like I know what I'm talking about, but in reality I'm pretty clueless about muscle names. Except glutes. Because that's just fun to say.)

4. NO CARDIO RECOMMENDATION. We stuck with our same cardio schedule—daily, with guilt—since we had no other guidance.

Overall, it's a good workout—plenty hard with nice variety. I'll definitely keep it on file for when I feel like changing stuff up. I particularly recommend it for lower body and core work.

Quiz Answer: "e"—all of the above.

We got asked that question at least five times a day, so we had ample opportunity to use all of those answers. The best response was when I said we were having an imaginary picnic, the woman asking didn't even blink before answering, "So what are you eating?" I guess crazy attracts crazy.

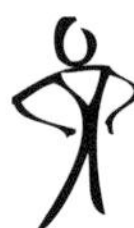

P·E·R·S·O·N·A·L·|·E·S·S·A·Y

On Medicating and Meditating

Oh, ohm already. Despite my many initial misgivings about meditation—what if I fail? At sitting! And thinking!—upon a friend's recommendation, I finally decided to give it a try. What I discovered is that meditation is a far more powerful tool than I previously ever gave it credit for. It helped me find a place of peace in myself that I didn't even know existed. But before I can begin to tell you about the finding, I must first tell you about the losing. Allow me to back up.

I am not a peaceful person.

I have been many things: Energetic, morose. Friendly, moody. Gregarious, overly sensitive. Dramatic, empathetic. But never peaceful. As my father put it, I'm a thrasher. It took me twenty-five years to figure out that not everyone walks around feeling like their skin is on wrong ways out. But as is often the case, that which we lack is what we need the most.

And so I have sought peace—and found it with varying degrees of success—in many different places over the years. In high school I was a mess. It's true. I was the class Valedictorian. But with ulcers and an eating disorder and, of all things, an illiterate boyfriend. One of the most common things people said to me then was, "Just when I think I get to know you, I realize I don't know anything about you at all." Which is because I didn't know anything about me. There was no peace for me in high school.

In college, I found a measure of peace in cognitive behavioral therapy and volunteering in the campus crisis center and dancing and a troupe of friends who managed to be both hilariously insane and functional. And then the Very Bad Boyfriend arrived to steal my fledgling sense of self and left me dashed on the rocks of my own self-doubt. Graduate school gave my manic energy an outlet but revived the ulcers and, unsupervised, took the eating disorder to a whole new level. This is also the time in my life where I first started having horrible panic attacks, later "diagnosed" (if one can really diagnose a syndrome) as Irritable Bowel Syndrome, that would send me to the hospital multiple times; my only complaint being that my body was trying to eat itself from the inside out. There was little peace for me in college.

After college there were many who worked hard to stabilize me. My life, as it has always been, was enacted against the ethereal backdrop of my LDS faith, bordered on each side by the tightly woven curtain of my family. Which is why it always pains me to talk of my deep sadness. Because it causes them to cry, "How did we fail you?" when the truth is that they never did. Well, no more than what is merely human, anyhow. The failing—or the falling—was all mine. It was my crazy whacked-out, high-strung self. Blame it on brain chemicals, hormones, genetics, or—my personal favorite—a deep-seated fatal flaw, but don't ever blame it on them.

It wasn't until the tailspin brought on by my first miscarriage and then the death of my first child, a daughter, Faith (also known as the reason why I often write I have birthed five children, and yet you'll only hear me talk about three cherubic boys and my darling daughter), that I ever considered medication. I don't even remember how the conversation came about—perhaps it is de rigueur for mothers of dead babies—but my family doctor gave me a prescription for Celexa. I took it. It made me dizzy. But it also evened me out. It didn't take much; I am what they consider a "responder" to medicine. One Vicodin renders me unconscious for six hours. Narcotics are so overwhelming to my system that I refuse to take them ever, for anything, even after childbirth. And so it was with the Celexa. Within a couple of months, I began to chafe at the chemical bonds that bound in my euphoria as much as they bound up my tears. I quit it cold turkey after three short months. Every medical professional will tell you that you are never to do this. I had a rough month or so, but then it was out and I was fine. And I was me again. I took up yoga to help quell the panic that had come back but, in my frenetic spirit, I only did the kind of yoga that made you sweat and shake and count your breaths in your head.

The next time I took an antidepressant was Wellbutrin. The need came after more than a year of caring for a dear family member with a chronic illness. In addition, I was overwhelmed after my third son's recent birth, sad to have recently moved, sad that it was winter. My gynecologist prescribed it for me. That was a mistake. Wellbutrin is not for people with a history of eating disorders. It is also not for people with anxiety problems. I took it for six months until I was so irritable that I irritated myself with how irritating I was. I went cold turkey. Again. Fortunately, for me anyhow, it was easy to stop taking it. I had no side effects. In fact, I immediately felt better. I was me again.

Third time's the charm, right? As part of my treatment for my compulsive over-exercising, I started taking Cymbalta—this time prescribed to me by an actual psychiatrist—to help with the anxiety brought on by the dark days and also to help ameliorate my compulsion to over-exercise. It helped. But I didn't like the side effects. After several months of going back and forth over the cost-benefit analysis of the meds, I decided it wasn't worth it. And did it again. Cold turkey. This time it was a total freaking rush. Two weeks of "brain shivers"—an event I can only describe as exactly that: as if my brain were shivering inside my skull. It isn't as unpleasant as it sounds. I got my energy back, my sex life improved, and my thoughts were no longer fragmented into a puff of paper snowflakes that swirled around me with every eddy, never settling and never coalescing. It was so great, I was tempted to go back on the Cymbalta just so I could have the pleasure of going off of it again.

So why do I tell you all this? Well, for one, I have a penchant for over-sharing. You may have noticed. But mostly I wanted to say that if there ever was a girl who needed meditation, it would have been me. In this time and this place. And I think it's working. I really do.

I lost no weight thanks to the meditating; nor did I have any life-changing epiphanies; and I had no better luck regulating my breathing while running through side stitches. But it gave me something better: the realization that I do have the potential—nay, even the ability—to be peaceful in myself. I will not say that I will never again need medication. I most likely will. And if that day comes, I will take it and be grateful. But the great thing is that I have the rest of my life to keep working on it.

chapter six

June
Jillian Michaels

WHILE ALL MY EXPERIMENTS ARE UNIQUE, this one had an element I had never before experienced and that threw me for a real loop: the inimitable Jillian Michaels. You think she drives you nuts on *The Biggest Loser*? Now you too can experience some of the yelling, crying, and all-around drama in the privacy of your own life, via her book, *Making the Cut* by Jillian Michaels (Three Rivers Press, 2008).

Before I started this Experiment, I had no particular feelings about Jillian. (Yeah, we're on a first-name basis. Just like Madonna and me. And Mr. Bimble, the man who lives in my finger.) Not being a TV watcher save for the occasional PBS documentary on food and/or eating disorders—it's sick, I know—to this day I've never seen a single episode of *The Biggest Loser*. Culturally irrelevant, that's me! And so I was blindsided by the force that is Jillian Michaels. Over the course of the month, my emotions swung wildly from major girlcrush to hater and then settling somewhere around dubious respect. I should have called this The Great PMS Experiment, my mood swings were that severe. That woman.

I am not the only one she does this to. The salesman at Barnes & Noble took one look at my purchase and said, "You're not going to do that are you? That chick is one scary dude." After I told him that I wanted to see what all the hype was about, he leaned conspiratorially over the counter and added, "Strong women can be a real bitch." In addition to being grammatically incorrect, his offensive opinion actually made me more excited to get home and get started. (Incidentally, the whole B&N experience made me wonder what he says to people who buy *How to Deal with Cat Fetishism.*)

The Theory

JILLIAN MICHAELS AND I SHARE A SIMILAR WEAKNESS: We're both research junkies. This predilection to let white-coated folks tell her what to do is manifest early on in her book. Right away, from page one, she's the tough-talking, no-excuses, drill-sergeant trainer that you—because you, being culturally in tune, have probably seen the show—have come to know and love. Or hate. Or love to hate. Or hate to love. (Seriously, I have never seen a personal trainer inspire such intense emotions in people!) She begins, "This book is not for the faint of heart. Over the next thirty days you are mine, and this is your bible. [. . .] This is not some namby-pamby "lifestyle" book that's going to waffle on about moderation for "better health" and leave you with the warm-fuzzies. It's about seeing how far you can go, getting a little crazy, and maybe along the way making that ex of yours want you back. The bottom line? It's about getting in the best shape of your life—so let's get ripped."

Okay, so we're not even going to pretend this is about better health, she refuses to coddle me and gives me permission to be crazy. I love her.

To show you how serious she is about her warning to the faint of heart among us, Jillian actually has a test at the beginning of her book that you must pass to continue with her program. Sheer marketing genius! First you tell a person that you will build them the body of their dreams and then you make it an exclusive club. I wanted in so badly that I did that test. Right there on my bedroom floor. In my Lucky Charms pajamas ($3.99 + one box top + $10.00 shipping and handling . . . hmmm) at 10:30 at night. I passed.

Are you cool enough to hang with Jillian and me? First you must be looking to only lose the last ten-to-twenty pounds of "vanity weight." Second, you have to have a "moderate" level of fitness, which she defines as being able to do the following:

> **1.** Step on and off a twelve-inch step for three minutes. Take your pulse for one minute. You need to be 119 or lower for women (107 for men).

2. Do as many push-ups ("Girly push-ups? I don't even want to hear it—toughen up or go buy someone else's book.") as you can in one minute. Women need twelve or more, men at least thirty.

3. Do as many sit-ups as you can in one minute. Twenty-five or more gets the women in, thirty-one gets the men.

4. Do a wall sit. Minimum of thirty seconds is required although sixty-to-ninety seconds is expected.

Raise your hand if you just had ugly flashbacks from the Presidential Fitness Challenge in middle school! The only thing missing was the sit-n-reach. I loved the sit-n-reach. I hated middle school.

Anyhow, the key component to this program is giving up control. Jillian is very upfront about wanting you to give her total control over your food, your workouts, and basically your entire life except for your boring, mundane job that you wouldn't have if your abs were as spectacular as hers (truly, I covet them). She wants you to trust her. I have a very hard time trusting fitness people. However, I also have a really hard time saying no to a challenge.

The Workout

THE BOOK DIVIDES THE WORKOUTS INTO TEN CIRCUITS made up of weights and HIIT (high-intensity interval training; read more about this in chapter 10). You do two circuits per week, each circuit is done for two days and must be completed in less than forty-five minutes. Yay, more circuit training! Additional cardio is up to you but must be done after her circuit. She requires you (yes, requires) to commit to exercising an hour a day, five days a week.

My first surprise of the book came when I discovered she schedules in rest days every Wednesday, Saturday, and Sunday. So this plan actually had Allison and I working out less than we usually do. But, perhaps sensing my encroaching dubiousness, she assured me that we would make up for it with intensity. And for all you smart alecks who are right now pointing out that 5+3=8 and not 7, let me clarify that she wants you to commit to working out five days a week. Her circuits only take up four days, so you have to come up with something on your own for the fifth day—probably some low-and-slow cardio.

The Food

JILLIAN'S WEIGHT/CARDIO CIRCUITS BEING FAIRLY MAINSTREAM, her diet—and I'm not even going to pretend it is anything other than a diet—is where the extremism comes in. It starts out with asking you to determine your "oxidation type," meaning how your body utilizes oxygen in burning food. You may not have known you were "oxidizing," as most people just mistake it for "breathing." Fools. Everyone's cells use oxygen to convert food into energy. This is called cellular oxidation. Back in the 1930s (incidentally, the era for best women's hats ever), while everyone else was worrying about how to procure food without resorting to the Joad method, scientists discovered that the rate at which people oxidize their food varies. Researchers postulated that given this natural variation, usually attributed to genetics and climate of origin, different types of oxidizers would thrive on different types of food.

According to *Making the Cut,* there are three basic types:

> SLOW OXIDIZERS: "Also known as carbo types or sympathetic dominant. They generally have relatively weak appetites, a high tolerance for sweets, problems with weight management, 'type A' personalities, and are often dependent on caffeine."
>
> BALANCED OXIDIZERS: "Mixed types are neither fast nor slow oxidizers, and are neither parasympathetic nor sympathetic dominant. They generally have average appetites, cravings for sweets and starchy foods, relatively little trouble with weight control, and tend towards fatigue, anxiety, and nervousness."
>
> FAST OXIDIZERS: "Also known as protein types or parasympathetic dominant. They tend to be frequently hungry, crave fatty, salty foods, fail with low-calorie diets, and tend towards fatigue, anxiety, and nervousness. They are often lethargic or feel 'wired,' 'on edge,' with superficial energy while being tired underneath."

According to Jillian, your oxidation type changes your macronutrient ratios. Specifically, slow oxidizers should eat Ornish at 60 carb/25 protein/15 fat. Balanced oxidizers go with The Zone at 40/30/30. Fast oxidizers are Atkins at 20/50/30. She then goes on to give you a complete list of foods in every category that you should and should not eat, depending on your type, complete with menus.

This was interesting to me because a) I covet Jillian's abs, and b) if I allow myself to eat how I feel best, I fall very close in line with her slow oxidizer recommendations, which according to her test, is what I am. Given the hype lately around low-carb and no-carb, I have tried to limit my carbs. This makes me feel groggy, lethargic, and all-around crappy (see the next chapter on the Primal Blueprint Experiment). But as soon as I get my carb infusion—usually via healthy foods like whole grains or fruit, although a bag of jelly beans will also do the trick—then I feel awesome again. I love it when research tells me what I want to hear! (And that part about being a Type A, caffeine-addicted psycho with weight-management issues? Yeah, I'll own that too. Sigh.)

In addition to eating for your oxidation type, Jillian also gives you a daily calorie recommendation. Are you ready for this? She expects you to survive and work out on your BMR (basal metabolic rate), which is the number of calories your body needs just to survive. The best way to determine your BMR is to do "metabolic testing" that involves sitting in a room and running on a treadmill with a gas mask hooked up to a computer strapped over your face. Which, take it from me (because you know I've tried it!) is only fun if you get your thrills from suffocating. Otherwise, there are a bunch of calculators out there to give you a good estimate. Once you know your BMR and your oxidation type, she has meals spelled out for you for the entire month. She even includes recipes!

Peak Week

Having heard body builders discuss the concept of "peaking," I was interested to discover that Jillian includes a chapter on how to get into peak form for a special event, using her photo shoot for the cover of the book as an example. Giving her props for honesty, I will tell you it involves tactics like caffeine pills, lengthy sauna trips, and treadmill runs in heavy clothing to sweat out extra water and extremely low-cal/low-carb diets (600 calories/day). She warns to only do it for a week to get in "peak" form. I would warn you to never do it. Ever. I get that fitness models and celebrities do this kind of nonsense, which is exactly why I'm glad I'm not one. The peak week chapter was one of the most interesting parts of her book to me, as it refutes all the crap that celebrities spew about eating whatever they want and only walking their dog for exercise to get in bikini shape. However, from a practical standpoint, it was also the least useful chapter for me.

In the Gym

NOT QUITE A WEEK INTO IT AND ALREADY THERE WAS CONFUSION. The Gym Buddies and I unanimously agreed that her circuits are too easy. I know! All that blather at the beginning about being in shape before starting and this book isn't for wusses, blah, blah, blah, and then you end up only having to hold your plank for ten seconds? Do not misunderstand: I am not super fit. I am of a fairly average fitness level. And yet not only are these workouts not challenging, but they're just not crazy. For the love of little green apples, we were promised crazy and we want to get crazy!

Jillian says the circuits should be done once through with no rest in between and should take you about forty-five minutes. They took us about twenty minutes the first day and thirty the next because we were trying hard to slow it down and really max out our reps. But, my excitement was restored when I realized that Jillian says you can do the circuits twice through if you want a more intense workout. After doubling up each circuit and upping the recommended weights, speeds, and inclines, it turned out to be a serious workout.

As for the diet part of it, that was disastrous. Part of it was my fault—I'd been trying to avoid grains for so long that apparently I didn't know how to eat them anymore and thereby messed up my macronutrient ratios. But part of it was the diet's fault—I can survive on my BMR, but I sure can't thrive! I hate feeling like I'm starving all the time. I suppose this is the part where Jillian would get all up in my grill and yell, "You want easy? Then go home! This isn't about easy!" and I'd break down and cry about how I hate my thighs and my life sucks (even though it doesn't) and then we'd cry and hug and I'd throw out my ice cream in dramatic fashion while the camera pans across my tear-stained face.

Yeah, well. I ate the ice cream. And I upped my calories to 1,500 a day. Theoretically, with all the workouts I do, I should still lose weight.

Out of the Gym

WANT TO GET PEOPLE ALL RILED UP at your next family reunion? (Nothing says family fun like family feud!) Ask them what they think of Jillian Michaels. It turns out that she—not President Clinton—is the great polarizing factor of this generation. Some people hate her, some think she's a goddess, but rarely will you find anyone who says, "Jillian? Meh." And like any good consumer in our culture, I began to have opinions about her too.

How She Eats

My first brush with the Jillian Phenomenon was in reading an interview on the Web site neversaydiet.com with Ali Vincent, the first woman to win *The Biggest Loser*. Ali gushed about working with the world's most famous personal trainer, "She is a great example of fulfilling your destiny. She'll order dessert and take one bite and then pour the salt shaker over it. She's about living consciously."

I take issue with anyone, celebrity or otherwise, talking about "living consciously" and "fulfilling your destiny" by manipulating your food. Your food is not your consciousness nor your destiny. Do you know why? Because your body is not the sum of your consciousness nor your destiny. We are more than what we eat. We are more than what we look like. (And if I say that enough times, one of these days I'm going to believe it, by golly.)

Several years ago when the media was all aflutter over "Pro-Ana" and "Pro-Mia" sites—a small subset of Web sites that enable girls in pursuing their disordered lifestyles—many eating disorder "tips" were published in the news. For those of us who already possessed the eating disordered mindset but up until then were blissfully unaware of such sites, this was like a gold mine. I'm not proud to admit it, but I spent a considerable amount of time on those Web sites. Mostly, they were not what the media portrayed them to be—i.e., fist pumping bastions of alternative lifestyles (die-styles?)—but rather collections of depressed, withdrawn, and highly competitive sick girls. Most of them (us?) didn't want to stay disordered forever. Most of us realized how much our eating disorder took from us. But all of us wanted to be thin. And so the site authors published tips and tricks for getting to that Waif Ideal.

Some tips were bizarre like the fabled and much reported "eat toilet paper because it fills you up and has no calories" one. I personally never knew anyone that did that or even said they did that, although apparently it had enough cultural cache to make it on a *Law & Order* episode. Other tips were painful, like swallowing cups of vinegar to take away your appetite (and your esophagus!) or punching yourself in the stomach to quell pesky hunger pangs. But there were quite a few tips that actually sounded a wee bit sensible, especially to a person desperate to lose weight. My favorite of those is the destroy-your-food tip.

In April of 2008 I was invited to be a guest on Fox's morning show, *The Mike and Juliette Show*, to talk about how girls learn disordered eating habits. The thing I remember most was the host Juliette—who was so thin herself that her chest bones were visible through her low-cut dress and then had the audacity to tell me that she simply couldn't understand why I ever had an eating disorder because she just "loves food too much!"—asking me about spraying Windex on a hamburger to keep myself from eating it. While that particular incident was not true (seriously, do these people not have cue cards for a reason?) as I was mostly a vegetarian, the general idea behind it was true.

When I was fifteen, I took an ill-advised job as a waitress for the catering department of the nearby university. Very quickly I discovered that not only was I younger and more naive (as evidenced by the fact that I did not wear a black or red bra peeking out under my white tuxedo shirt) than most of my fellow waitresses, but I was also, well, chubbier. At least to my eyes. In a profession that relies heavily on being attractive to make money, the svelte sylphs I worked with soon became my idols.

Due to the above-par talent of the chefs, we were constantly surrounded by an array of rich and delicious foods. Yes, we had to serve the dreaded and nasty "pasta bar" on more occasions than I care to remember, but there was always something fattening and exquisite to be had back in the kitchens. The temptation of the meltaway cookies was great for me. But so was my desire to be accepted. And so I watched those girls very carefully to see how they maintained their figures.

They destroyed their food.

Sometimes that entailed drowning it in an incompatible or extreme flavor—like salad dressing on cheesecake, raw horseradish layered on crème brulee, or even, like Jillian, the contents of the salt shaker poured out over a fifty-dollar plate of prime rib. Other times it meant "accidentally" spilling cleaning fluid on the leftover butterflake rolls or squirting dish soap into a chafing dish of hollandaise sauce. The entire goal was to make your plate of food as unappealing as possible. We didn't hide it. In fact, it became a game. The mealtime sport was who could eat the least dinner (and drink the most Diet Coke!) at dinner time.

And so it was with this background that I read this "diet tip" from the famed trainer-to-the-hoi-polloi. Not only do I take issue with the blatant wastefulness of the gesture—"Look! I can afford to pay $17.95 for a decadent piece of gourmet restaurant cake *and* I am so wealthy that I can afford to take one bite and then render the rest inedible."—but I am also offended by what this says about our bodies. To me, this displays an inherent distrust of your body. It makes it so that you treat your body as if it were an enemy to be conquered, subdued, or tricked rather than what it is—your ultimate partner in your health and well-being.

If all Jillian really wants is one bite of cake, then why not instruct her server to only bring her one bite of cake? (Oh, they'll do it! Especially if she's still paying full price for it.) Or why doesn't she split the piece with the whole table? Everyone gets a bite. Instead she perpetuates a method of disordered eating that, frankly, is a very slippery slope. What's next? Chewing and spitting? Eating food out of the garbage can that you threw away in an attempt to make it inedible?

It's taken me a lot of years to learn that food is a gift. It is not something to be feared or demonized but rather to be eaten with joy and thanksgiving. Take it from someone who has eaten food out of the garbage.

How She Looks

In addition to having an opinion about how she treats food, suddenly I found myself having an opinion on how she looks. While the former put me firmly in the hater camp, the latter definitely had me girlcrushing again. And I'm not the only one with opinions about her physique. The number one comment I got from people both in real life and on my Web site during this Experiment was about how she looks. Opinions ranged from people thinking she looked like a dude all the way to people worshipping her bufftastic abs in complicated ceremonies. See what I mean about her? Drama!

No matter what you think of Jillian now, you have to admit she has made an incredible physical transformation. Judging from past pictures and from her own reports, she was no genetically blessed wunderkind like so many of our celebrities (*cough*Gwyneth Paltrow*cough*). She has worked long and hard to get where she is and you have to admire that in a person.

All of this body-ideal talk got me thinking. Back in the day, when I started my whole fitness kick (What—you thought I was always this crazy?), I was the softest, squishiest geek you ever pushed into her high school locker. Amy Lee of Evanescence—yes, I went through a Goth phase, and, yes, I know I just dated myself, shut UP and let me finish already—was my ideal body type, and I thought that Kelly Ripa looked "hard," with her visible pecs and bulging bis.

And so it was with this attitude that I found Tom Venuto's book *Burn the Fat, Feed the Muscle,* which became my weight lifting and nutrition bible for the next year. The subtitle read: *How to be a fitness model or just look like one.* At the time, I thought the term "fitness model" meant the girls who appear in *Shape* and *Self* and other fitness magazines. Who wouldn't want to look like that? It was a couple of years before I realized that "fitness model" is an actual title that means something far more muscular (and tanned) than those skinny girls.

But by then I was too firmly ensconced in the fitness world to care. I loved my exercise. I loved my new muscles. I loved that I could climb up the fireman pole at the playground *without using my legs*. I loved that when I flexed my back, it actually rippled. And it never occurred to me that I had passed right on by Amy Lee and was closing in on Kelly Ripa, although I'll never have her abs—but it's not for lack of trying.

The change was subtle. Slowly but surely, I started thinking of starlets like Kirsten Dunst and Mischa Barton and Lindsay Lohan as "squishy" and "untoned" and even "skinny fat." Theirs was no longer a body ideal I aspired to. But I didn't really realize how far I'd come until a good friend's husband looked at my Jillian Michaels book and wrinkled his nose, "What girl would want abs like that? Gross!" Me, apparently.

The Results

MY RESULTS WERE UNIMPRESSIVE. This could be due to the fact that while I ate her prescribed foods for the month, I did not adhere to her caloric restrictions. However, my real feeling is that neither the workout nor the diet is particularly revolutionary. The strength of this program lies in Jillian's considerable charisma. If you love her particular brand of drill sergeant/therapist/celebrity mojo, then this program may work better for you. But since none of the Gym Buddies showed any results either, I'm guessing it's the kind of thing that's better done in person.

What I Liked

FIRST AND FOREMOST, I loved her honesty about how hard she and other Hollywood types work for their physiques. I also loved her no-nonsense, no-coddling tone. In addition, her workouts were solid. You can tell that this is her field of expertise as this was the real strength of the book. And, since I now own the book, I will probably continue to use some of her workouts (slightly adapted, natch) to break up my routine.

What I Didn't Like

THE FOOD PLAN. Problemo numero uno: the insanely low daily calorie allotment. She expected me to not only wake up every morning and take care of my house and kids but to *work out* on my BMR: a measly 1,300 calories a day. Even refugee camps provide 1,800. And then there was the issue of the food itself. It tasted terrible. Every recipe I tried turned out badly although that could be chalked up to my lack of kitchen skillz. I was also bothered by the overabundance of mercury-contaminated large fish on the menu (one day in my menu plan called for six ounces of swordfish followed up the next day with the same—the FDA recommends avoiding swordfish altogether, as it is one of the most heavily contaminated fish in the ocean.)

I also have to say that I will not miss her smirk on her cover photo. Seriously, after a few days I started turning it over just so she'd stop looking at me like that. Jillian can kick my butt in the gym any day, but she can't make me dinner after.

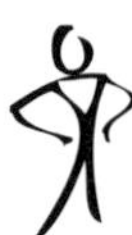

Best Moment

All my crazy finally paid off with the aforementioned trip to New York City to be on The Morning Show with Mike and Juliette. *While doing the the show itself sucked—any of you interested in being on a reality TV show have more cajones than I do—the fun part was that they flew me and my sister Laura out to New York City and put us up in a fancy hotel for two days. Having eight kids between the two of us and living several states apart, we barely get to talk on the phone uninterrupted, much less have two days in one of the greatest cities on earth all to ourselves. Laura and I could have fun kicking pebbles down a dirt road, so turning us loose in NYC was a dream come true. It was a fabulous—and free!—vacation that ended up being one of the best memories of my adult life. Sure, you know NYC has Broadway and Fifth Avenue and all those shiny lights in Times Square, but did you know they also have the best vegetarian buffet ever and a Naked Cowboy to go with it?! That's right, he marches around in nothing but his boots and a pair of tighty-whities toting his guitar and—the best part—getting tourists to pay him to take pictures of him grabbing their butts. It's like a Fulbright Scholarship for frat boys. Only in America.*

P·E·R·S·O·N·A·L·|·E·S·S·A·Y

The Biggest Loser Reinforces Gender Stereotypes

QUESTION: If you could do one exercise for the rest of your life, what would it be? Why?

JILLIAN MICHAELS: Running because—although I hate it—it's most effective at making my butt smaller.

BOB HARPER: I love to run so it would be that. It is a great cardiovascular exercise and a great calorie burner.

In this 2008 interview sponsored by Oprah and, ironically, Hersheys, both of *The Biggest Loser* trainers give the same answer—running—and yet for wildly different reasons. The female trainer would run even though she has said time and again that she hates it. With all the exercises out there to choose from, why would she condemn herself to an eternity doing the one that she despises? Because it makes her butt smaller. Apparently, hell is treadmills and skinny jeans with no Spanx.

On the other hand, the male trainer not only picks what he loves doing, but he does it because primarily it will strengthen his cardiovascular system and enhance his long-term health prospects.

Jillian Michaels is exceptionally dedicated. She has already proven her will to lose weight and her willpower to keep it off at all costs. According to all the statistics, she is an aberration, albeit the aberration we all wish we were. But what of the rest of America, as in the women who sit in their living rooms and watch *The Biggest*

Loser? What kind of message about exercise does it send to them and to their young daughters who are also watching and learning about what it means to be a girl?

To me it says that exercise is to be hated but must be done anyhow because you are nothing if you have a big butt.

On my Web site, I asked my readers why they exercise. The results were close, with 35 percent of the nearly 700 respondents answering, "Yeah, I say it's primarily about my health, but I love that it makes me look better too." While 29 percent answered, "It's mostly about my looks—the health benefits are just an added bonus." (The remaining 36 percent were divided between an assortment of other witty responses.) I'm wondering now how it would have panned out if I had asked people to specify their gender.

I am inclined to posit that the trainers on *The Biggest Loser* are representative of our society as a whole. That men are more inclined to think of exercise in terms of its salutatory benefits—and thereby are more likely to make it a lifelong endeavor—while women are taught to think of it in terms of our, ahem, *bottom line.* Most men will continue their weekly pick-up games even if their waistline doesn't shrink because they are having fun reliving high school glory days and smacking each other on the rear (not really socially acceptable in the office.) While many women will opt to do a form of exercise they don't necessarily enjoy (anyone else see the stepmill as a modern-day Sisyphus parallel?) and then give up in frustration when the desired proportions are not achieved. Studies have shown that people who exercise primarily for their looks are more likely to get discouraged quickly and less likely to stick with it over the long term.

In addition to the message perpetuated by Jillian Michaels—who at least works out—women are also treated to the alternate Hollywood view of exercise, courtesy of Alessandra Ambrosio, Victoria's Secret model and mother of then three-month-old Anja. When asked how she regained her world-famous body so quickly after childbirth, she replied, "I only do yoga once a week or so, but that's it for now." So exercise is to be endured in order to gain a svelte figure. Unless it doesn't work and then you should sue your parents for losing you the genetic lottery. Now I'm depressed.

Which is probably why Hershey's sponsored the interview.

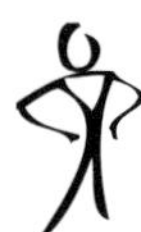

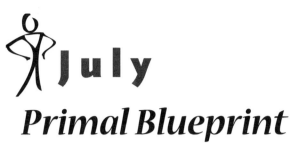

chapter seven

July
Primal Blueprint

I'M A VEGETARIAN who likes long runs in the woods and fine chocolate. He was a Neanderthal who dined on raw meat, plants, and grubs and only ran when chased by a ravenous predator. You'd think I would have known better than to go out with a Workout I only met over the Internet. But then you'd also think I would have known better than to lock myself on a roller coaster on a dare. I had to ride that sucker for a full forty-five minutes before they could find the manager to get me out. The moral of this story: I am not known for my common sense.

It all began, like most of my Experiments, with a Web site. I've never met a fitness book, article, or site that I haven't immediately devoured, and this one was no different. It seduced me with promises of hard-core workouts, healthy meals, and eye-popping results in a short amount of time, all standard wooing techniques in this industry. But The Primal Blueprint by Mark Sisson (www.marks dailyapple.com), developed by former elite triathlete Mark Sisson, took me one better—it actually had research backing its claims.

I read along for months, trying a recipe here and there, reading every new research tidbit with gusto and occasionally trying out various aspects of the program, but I couldn't fully commit to the program. Until the fateful day they said the magic words to me: "We challenge you." I might as well have been fourteen years old at the amusement park again. I cannot turn down a good challenge. And so I signed on.

One month to eat, drink, and be merry like our pre-agrarian ancestors. Clubbing and hair-dragging would be optional, I presumed. Yes, it was going to be a big change. But, hey, big changes often yield big results. Or big meltdowns.

The Theory

THE PRIMAL BLUEPRINT IS A RETURN TO SIMPLER TIMES. Much simpler. Since there was no farming back in the prominent-brow-ridge days, humans had to rely on whatever they could kill or pull from the dirt. They were doing the 100-mile diet long before anyone knew what a mile was.

The Diet

No grains. Grains are poison. I think that pretty much sums it up. Neanderthals like simple sentences as well as simple food, apparently. If you want more detail, try to keep your carbohydrates at or below 100 grams a day and get the majority of those carbs from a variety of fruits and vegetables. But don't get too fond of the food because millions of years ago the food supply was anything but stable. So in addition to knowing what you can and can't eat, you should also plan for a few days of intermittent fasting (primal code for not eating).

Yes, Please

Eat as many veggies as you want. Watch the starchy ones like potatoes, peas, and carrots though, so you stay under that arbitrary 100g of carbs per day.

Fat is your new best friend. And the primal folk don't care about it being saturated or high in cholesterol either, for which they have some science-y reasoning that probably just made the American Heart Association throw up a little. Load up on nuts (but not peanuts as they are technically a legume and not a nut), fry your eggs in butter, and go to work licking the steak grease off your fingers. Grew up in the fat-phobic '90s like I did? Try not to hyperventilate, the panic will subside.

The last Primal staple is flesh. They don't specify, but I'm assuming Grok—their cutesy moniker for the typical Neanderthal—wouldn't differentiate between humans and animals. All I'll say is that you should obey local laws. So unless you are stranded on an

Andean mountain peak or your last name is Donner, you'd better stick to loads of fish, seafood, poultry, pork, and beef. Don't worry about it being lean. Suck the marrow out of the bones and eat the organs if it makes you happy. Hard-core Primals go raw, even. Being a long-time vegetarian, this was the scariest part of the experiment for me.

In Moderation

Go easy on the fruit.

For the thirty-day Experiment, they recommended going full bore and avoiding all dairy, although they do say that once you are at a happy weight and body fat percentage, it's okay to have a little of the high-quality stuff like cottage cheese or Greek yogurt every now and then. The weekend before I started my new Primal lifestyle included a little cheese-going-away party. As I discovered during my Vegan Experiment, I can do without drinking milk just fine. I can also live without "chunk cheese." But I truly mourned the temporary loss of my Greek yogurt and double-cream brie.

Also, try to limit the beans. I know they keep you regular but they're high in carbs and have something scary in them called an anti-nutrient, which might be one of the most awesome pseudoscience words I've ever read.

No, Thank You

No sugar. Oh, come on, you knew that one was coming! It's the simplest carb there is! And of course you know alcohol is a sugar, right? Also, no grains or anything made from grains—not even the all-mighty whole grains. By the way, corn is a grain and not a vegetable.

This Is Not Atkins

Besides the no-dairy policy, the Primal Diet places an emphasis on eating foods as our ancestors did. It isn't enough that something is "low carb"—it needs to be quality, real food. Protein bars are a big no-no. Primal eaters are especially concerned with the quality of meat, urging everyone to eat grass-fed and finished beef, wild-raised and caught fish, and, of course, organic and locally grown fruits and veggies. Yes, they suffer from the same California delusion about food as the rest of that state, so the rest of us will just have to do our best to keep things as natural as possible.

The Workout

IN A NUTSHELL: CROSSFIT. (See chapter 3.) According to the Primal Blueprint, cavemen worked out by walking long distances slowly interspersed with the occasional all-out run-ma-the-puma's-coming maximal sprint. They recommend throwing in the low kind of cardio, such as a nice meander through the underbrush, whenever you feel like it (don't forget to check for ticks!) with the sprints two-to-three times per week for about ten minutes. Grok would also have heaved a lot of heavy stuff around. So do weight training but make it heavy and make it functional (see chapter 1).

The Gym Buddies and I decided to stick with CrossFit as it covers the weights and the sprinting, so we don't have to think too much about it all. But, in our first fit of rebellion, we decided to keep our hip-hop dance class and kickboxing. I'm sure Grok danced. Mating ritual, anyone? And he'd definitely need the boxing, especially if that date ended badly.

Sundries

In addition to exercising like your day job consists of fire building, mating, and picking your teeth, true Primal Blueprint followers follow Grok's cue on personal hygiene. So here's your chance to get all Matthew McConaughey up in here and avoid deodorant, use only natural soaps and—I'm not kidding—take cold showers. What, you think Grok had a water heater? Move to the Amazon, wuss.

Strangely, they make no mention of dressing in loin cloths or carrying weapons in public places, but the Primal folk definitely endorse going barefoot when possible. If you can't go barefoot, then they encourage you to wear "anti-shoes" like Vibram FiveFingers.

In the Gym

AS MANY CHRONIC DIETERS KNOW, the first week on any program is the honeymoon week. If that were true, then Grok only sprang for two days in his great-aunt's rodent-infested cabin with me. It was one long week. I'll give you the good news first: Not a single grain crossed my lips for eight days. In addition, I single-handedly kept the raw nut industry in the black. Surprisingly, my intense CrossFit workouts did not suffer for lack of grains. I enjoyed CrossFit this time around just as much as the first—which is to say I hated every second of doing it, but I loved the results. Also good: no jelly beans, ice cream, candy, cookies, or any other sugary nonsense, which is even more impressive considering what time of the month it was. I honestly felt like I had more energy and was more stable without the White Satan.

Staying true to the Primal Blueprint, I included one day of intermittent fasting in the form of no food for twenty-four hours. I'd be all proud about that except that I'm used to it seeing as I'm LDS (aka "Mormon") and it's part of my religion. So I've been doing that part of the plan for years now.

I did cheat, however. While I had no problem giving up the moo juice, it ended up being too much to kiss all my beloved dairy good-bye. So I made a concession and allowed myself one Greek yogurt a day, which sadly became the highlight of my Paleo culinary experience. It was also a rough transition from full-veg to full-meat. I only ate meat once and wanted to throw up for hours afterward. The worst part was the sticker shock when buying my grass-fed, organic dead animals.

On the carb front, I will confess, I OD'ed on the fruit. Since I couldn't eat grains or sugar and my CSA (community-supported agriculture) gave me a delicious basket of picked-that-day organic peaches, plums, and melons, I had a week-long fruit binge. In the end though I still managed to keep my carbs under 100g per day. Grok gave me a high-five before wandering back to twiddle his new opposable thumbs.

Now for the bad news: I gained two pounds. Despite trying to be all enlightened and pretend that my weight does not define my worth as a woman, this development did not please me. Especially as I was hoping to lose the nine pounds from the overtraining debacle (see chapter 2) that were still clinging to my thighs. However, I couldn't blame the Paleo diet solely for this as there were, like I mentioned, girly hormonal issues at work this week.

Next week I will have to cut out the yogurt (sigh . . .), about half the fruit, and probably some of the nuts as well if I want to start seeing results. Seriously, I ate so many nuts that squirrels were giving me support-group pamphlets.

The halfway point of the Primal Blueprint Experiment found me trying to retain my good cheer, but it was getting increasingly harder. Everyone says that it gets easier the longer you do something, but that was not holding true for me. I still didn't like eating meat. I still missed my morning oatmeal and dark chocolate. The one ray of light was, due to all the veggies, I was not at all constipated. (Don't pretend you don't care about my bowels!)

Out of the Gym

THE DECLINE STARTED WITH A SEEMINGLY INNOCENT CAMPING TRIP. I did all right eating like Caveman Grok until I decided to live like Grok. My husband, having a natural Grok-like affinity for firebuilding and rock throwing, decided it would be fun if he and I took the kidlets (like Chiclets, but for bears) camping. Being the eternal optimist that I am, I thought it would be the perfect occasion to go full-bore Primal. Apparently the Minnesota State Parks & Rec folk agreed with me as they gave us the campsite farthest from the Port-a-Potties. I tell you, it doesn't get more Neanderthal than pooping on a big pile of other people's poop. Which, having three preschoolers, meant we made that long trek to the "stinky place" at least two million times a day and night.

The campground also had a lovely river, picnic tables, and a playground—all at least a half a mile away. I ate it up. I walked everywhere, toting a kid on each hip National Geographic style (but with my shirt on, thank you very much). I even got a nice long hike with one of my best girl friends, where we talked in the way that only people who are already deeply in tune with the other's brand of crazy can do. The coup d'etat was carrying a thirty-pound bundle of firewood on my head—ta-da!—from the ranger station to the campsite.

But if my living and exercise patterns followed Grok, my eating approximated Chris Farley. The result of all that fabulous exercise and fresh air was an appetite like a freaking raptor. Two clean weeks of no carbs combined with hunger like I hadn't experienced since pregnancy "made me" eat a Dairy Queen Chocolate Extreme Blizzard every day made for a three-day-long binge. I was so starved for carbs that I ate things I would never imagine eating before. I had Raisin Bran (I hate raisins!), white pancakes with fake syrup (I hate white flour and corn syrup!), Little Debbie snack cakes (I hate women named Debbie! Kidding!), gummy bears, Dutch oven cobbler, chips, soda, and pretty much anything else that couldn't run away from me. Luckily, the children are fast.

It was ugly. I've never in my life binged like that before. Even now I shudder remembering it.

Do cavewomen cry? The carb binge left me feeling like the trip was a personal failure. For the first time ever during an Experiment, I considered quitting before the month was over. I hate to quit things. I am as stubborn as they come. There were only two more weeks. And I really wanted this to work!

Week Three

I quit.

The Results

I CAN CATEGORICALLY SAY THAT THE PRIMAL BLUEPRINT was a spectacular failure. My only comfort was that if I was going to go down, at least I went down in a blaze of glory. Or Little Debbie ignominy. Whatever.

The Food Plan

I should have known better than to mess with my food. After years of living in this body, you'd think I would have learned to trust it over what someone else tells me it needs. I like being vegetarian. And it turns out I had a lot of reasons besides my health for not eating that much meat. I feel good eating some grains. While I do understand, courtesy of the legion of very vocal Primal fans that wrote me over the course of the month, that the Primal Blueprint's low-carb, high-fat plan works really well for a lot of people, it didn't work for me. I felt like crap on it. I seem to need some carbs to help me regulate my mood. Perhaps, if I'd been able to stick with it the whole month, my body would have acclimated, but two-and-a-half weeks of being an exhausted, cranky wench was enough for me.

I should also have known that any diet that requires strict restriction triggers my disordered eating. I felt like the dangerous combination of "righteous restricting" and "evil bingeing" was putting me dangerously close to eating disorder land. The end result was several weeks of full-on crazy and a promise to my therapist to not do any more Experiments that require huge changes in my eating.

I did learn some really good things though. I decided to continue to incorporate some meat, especially fish, into my diet on a semi-regular basis, thereby becoming what I describe as a "vegaquarian"—although all the cool kids are saying "flexitarian" these days. I also learned to be better about planning my meals around the vegetables first. And, of course, I loved the "cleanness" of it all and the whole foods emphasis.

The Exercise

Going back to CrossFit was like the New Kids On the Block reunion—fun, nostalgic, and made me feel like I was twelve again. However, the songs got old, and after doing it for a month, I remembered the little things that bug me (like Joey's falsetto!).

Another issue I had this time around was bulking up. I know, I know, girls can't bulk out from weight lifting. Here's the thing: Girls may not bulk up like men, seeing as we have so much less testosterone, but girls can get bulkier than they like to be. I know that for some people, bigger is always better. I am not afraid of

Worst Moment

All the carb restrictions took me to a new low: distracting my toddler with a garbage truck so I could sneak a bite of his PB&J (because everyone knows that it doesn't count if nobody sees you eat it, right?). I also ate fishy crackers off the floor. But what I hated most was telling Mark Sisson—who had been nothing but super nice and supportive—that I had utterly failed on his plan. I wanted to be a primal success story, I really did! And I hate disappointing people. But there you have it.

some muscle, but I like my legs to look lean and toned. Not Olympic Weight Lifter Barbie. And I gained two inches on my thighs.

The last problem was wrist pain. I forgot how joint intensive, especially in the wrists, CrossFit is. I'm already crippled that way from all the typing!

Conclusion

DISASTER ON ALL FRONTS. Weight gained. Fat gained. Inches gained. Mind lost. Sigh.

I think my friend Kevin said it best: "I think your Experiment has been a success. You've shown that this doesn't work for you, and you've done it in only two weeks! That's half the time it usually takes for you to decide something doesn't work, right? So all you've really done is save time. Great job. I'm impressed."

So this month I learned that I am not a slow learner!

P·E·R·S·O·N·A·L·|·E·S·S·A·Y

Control Freak

Be water.

This was the advice given me by a good friend—by good friend I mean that, while we share a half dozen LinkedIn connections and comment on each others kids' pictures on Facebook, we haven't actually spoken in five years. He is a second-degree black belt in Aikido. "Be water" was his sensei's motto. My friend had it tattooed down the back of his neck.

Back when we shared a workout plan (but different visions), every time I would struggle in the gym, get frustrated, lose my temper, and even cry occasionally, he would point to his neck. His version of Talk To The Hand. Then I would get irritated and accuse him of getting things too easily, of never having to struggle. Because I never saw him struggle. A successful, competitive body builder with a physique most men would kill for, things did seem to come naturally for him—at least in the gym. And in my narrow vision, which I charitably attribute to the follies of youth, I assumed that meant he didn't know pain. In spite of the fact that he emigrated here from a country known for its human-rights abuses. A country in which he still had a child. A country to which he would one day return, not out of compulsion but because he thought he could do more good for his people there than from here.

I remember one day as he watched me fail early on a weight set that I could usually do easily. I tried over and over again, each time more determined to meet my weight. Each time failing earlier and faster. Finally, it was apparent to even my sweat-stung eyes that I was achieving nothing. I whined. He stopped me with, "Why do you keep hitting the rocks? Just flow around them. Be water."

I did not learn how to be water then.

Aikido, of which I took exactly one semester in college and then quit because rolling endlessly across the floor made me dizzy (official reason) and because I wasn't progressing very quickly despite trying very hard (real reason), is a martial art defined by its passivity. It is an almost entirely defensive practice. Where Karate kicks and Tae Kwon Do blocks, Aikido just . . . flows. Like water. The key, so my sensei told me, was to use your opponent's energy against him. To keep as much of your own energy in reserve as possible. Which is why it hardly looked like his tiny five-foot-seven-inch form was moving while his six-foot opponent was flying across the room.

One evening, against his advice, I tried to copy him. Encouraging my reluctant (and much larger) opponent to come at me, I attempted to throw him, only to throw myself to the mat instead. It knocked the wind out of me. When I regained my senses, it was to the laughter of my classmates as my sensei pointed out my critical mistake: I was still holding the hand of my opponent. "Charlotte," he chided gently, "you have to learn to let go."

I did not learn how to let go then.

My father tried to teach me this lesson one night as he held my hand, my body convulsing in pain. I was in my last semester of graduate school, had just had a miscarriage, and then out of the blue was laid flat by unpredictable attacks of horrible pain. I couldn't eat. I couldn't sleep. I was sure it was something horrible like stomach cancer. My doctors thought it was heartburn. The answer was more psychological than either of us thought. We finally named it Irritable Bowel Syndrome—a label which gave me no comfort because while the pain was real, the treatment wasn't. It was just a syndrome after all, one probably brought on by too much stress. They gave me some pain pills to take when it got really bad that I avoided because the narcotics made me loopy (official reason). And they were suppositories (real reason).

Instead, I would crouch in a darkened bathroom, my intestines turning on themselves with worry, the peristalsis working against itself until the pain culminated in diarrhea, vomiting, or both. And then I could go to sleep. It got to be a vicious cycle: The fear of having "an attack" would bring one on, and then the pain would plant the seed of fear for the next time. Truly, those talking stomach commercials you see for Zelnorm are to IBS what elves are to Mordor.

It was during one of those crying-shaking moments when my dad sat on the floor and held my hand telling me, "If you can just stop thrashing . . . all your life you've been a thrasher. But it just muddies the water. If you could just hold still, all the silt would settle down, and you'd be able to see the bottom clearly."

I did not learn how to be still then.

There were too many unknowns. Would I graduate? If I did, what would I do without the comforting confines of academia? Would I ever have a child? Get a job? Would I have to move? Where?

But despite the giant unanswered question that was my life, now I knew that if I didn't learn this lesson, then the pain would hit and hit hard. It's incredibly motivating, pain. Slowly, I learned to make environmental changes to help my IBS. I limited fatty foods; I practiced yoga regularly with an emphasis on the yogic breathing cycle. But I still believed that there wasn't a problem out there that couldn't be solved by just trying harder.

Honestly, I've never been good at being mellow. I'm high-strung. Tightly wound. Over eager. Passionate. I try too hard. I overcompensate. I flail. I kick against the pricks. The problem with being a control freak though is that eventually the pressure becomes too immense and you crack under the weight of all the expectations you heap on yourself. When this happens to me, I go down hard. I fight and fight (or run and run), and then when I have no energy left, I cry and cry. When that is over, and I'm completely spent, I experience one of those rare moments of thoughtful stillness. And so it was tonight. Life has a way of reteaching you important lessons until you learn them.

Sometimes the hardest thing to do is to do nothing at all. Be water.

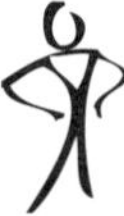

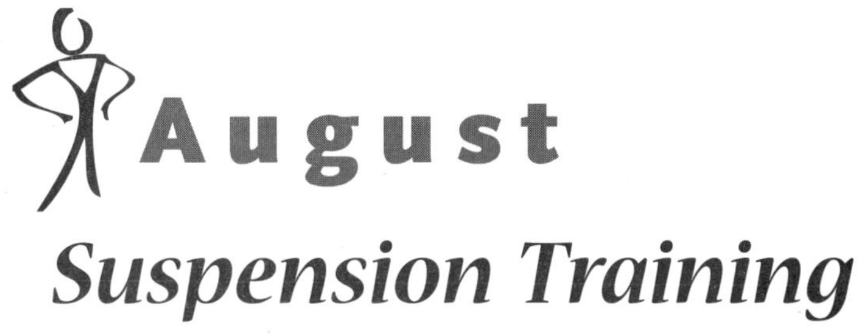

chapter eight

August
Suspension Training

"Just hanging around the gym, huh?"

"You swing by to say hello?"

"Your OB/GYN called—she wants her stirrups back."

"Me Tarzan. You Jane. Niiiice vine!"

"When you gonna do an iron cross?"

And my favorite . . . "You brought your sex swing to the gym?"

Bad puns, gynecological humor, sex jokes—just another inappropriate day at the gym courtesy of the smart alecks I work out with. It's even better when you consider that I go at 9:30 in the morning when my fellow gym goers are either moms of small kids like me, geriatric, or unemployed. Or possibly, just out of prison. (There is that one guy who uses a thick metal chain to tie a forty-five-pound weight plate to his torso before doing triceps dips. The plate dangles between his legs and clanks so ominously that Jacob Marley gets jealous.)

So what was it that elicited this latest round of one-liners? The Great Fitness Experiment for August was suspension training, which is exactly like it sounds: We trained whilst suspended. I had finally found The Great Workout in the Sky courtesy of a set of straps with handles and, yes, stirrups.

The Theory

BODYWEIGHT EXERCISES, OR MOVES THAT USE ONLY a person's body weight for resistance, are the oldest and most versatile exercises there are. All the old standbys like squats, lunges, push-ups, pull-ups, sit-ups, and all their attendant variations are considered bodyweight exercises. "The Prison Workout"—so named because prisoners can do it in its entirety within the confines of a tiny cell—is one popular example of a bodyweight-only workout.

The upside of this type of workout is that it can be done anywhere, anytime, and requires no equipment beyond your body. The downside? It's really boring. Sure, you can spice things up by adding plyometrics like squat jumps and jumping lunges; or you can combine exercises like burpees, the Devil's spawn of the squat thrust, the push-up, and the jump. But eventually people start wanting some variety and unless you really are a prisoner, then you are entitled to some variety.

The other concern people have with bodyweight exercises, aside from the lack of assortment, is that they tend to require high volume, and this makes people ask whether or not you can get a really good workout and build serious muscle using only your body. There is a school of thought—the lift-heavy-and-short methodology (see CrossFit and *Body for Life* for two examples)—that claims real muscle can only be built with lifting weights heavy enough to reach failure within ten-to-twelve reps. The only way to get that kind of weight is by pumping the iron.

This month, the Gym Buddies and I decided to test out this claim by doing only bodyweight exercises for a month. However, since we do like our entertainment, we used a device called a TRX to enable us to do a wider range of bodyweight exercises by adding suspension to the equation. Fitness Anywhere, the proprietors of the TRX, claim that you can get just as good of a workout using suspension training as you can by banging 'bells. All of which is to say we spent the month of August working out by hanging in the air.

I will say this: Never before nor since have I done an Experiment that has elicited so many comments from the peanut gallery.

The Workout

THE TRX IS A PRE-FAB CONTRAPTION consisting of two black nylon straps hanging from a tether. Each strap has a handle/stirrup on the end. You use it by simply attaching it to something taller than you—a ceiling beam, a door frame, Yao Ming—and then adjusting the handles/stirrups to different heights to facilitate a variety of exercises.

If you do not have access to a TRX and lack the 200 or so dollars that they retail for, there is no need for teeth gnashing or shirt rending. You can get easy-to-follow instructions on the Internet on how to construct your very own suspension trainer for about fifty dollars. It won't be as slick or as easily adjustable as the TRX, but then again it probably also won't get mistaken for a sex swing. Unless you're craftier than I think.

For our Experiment, we kept our cardio workouts the same and subbed in the suspension workouts for our weight training three days a week. No dumbbells or barbells or iron of any kind for an entire month! Thanks to the TRX's cushy handles, I didn't even need my cute little weight gloves that make me feel all hard-core even when I'm only lifting ten pounders. The TRX came with a total body workout, and so we started the first week with this basic routine:

1. Single Leg Squat
2. Balance Lunge
3. Hamstring Curl
4. Hip Abduction
5. Chest Press
6. Back Row
7. "Y" Shoulder Raise
8. Bicep Curl
9. Tricep Press
10. Supine Pull Through
11. Oblique Leg Raise
12. Suspended Crunch

If you don't know what some of these exercises are, no worries. There are plenty of video demos on the TRX Web site and other places on the Web. You can also use the suspension trainer for any type of exercise you would normally do, such as rows, squats, push-ups, pull-ups, etc. Even if you don't have access to a suspension trainer, you can still do some of the same exercises by looping a jump rope or resistance band around something sturdy. Just be careful not to let go and inadvertently shoot yourself across the room like a human cannonball. There are hundreds of variations, limited only by your imagination (just keep it legal, people).

In addition to strength moves, the suspension trainer can also be used for Pilates-like core work and facilitated stretching. Over the course of the month, I brought in new exercises to try nearly every day just so we could get a good idea of all the different ways suspension training could be used.

In The Gym

REALLY THIS SECTION SHOULD BE TITLED "Compromising Positions in the Gym" because, as we quickly discovered, it is very difficult to do suspension training and maintain one's dignity—at least at the beginning when you're still trying to learn all the moves. Thankfully a lifetime of embarrassing moments has conditioned me to survive—nay, embrace—public humiliation. It's hard to describe exactly how absurd we looked, and so I present to you the photographic evidence (see figure A).

(Note to self: Shorts were a bad idea. As were shoes. And pride.)

Setting up the TRX proved a bit tricky. It's simple as pie to swing it over an immovable object—the chin-up bar/cable

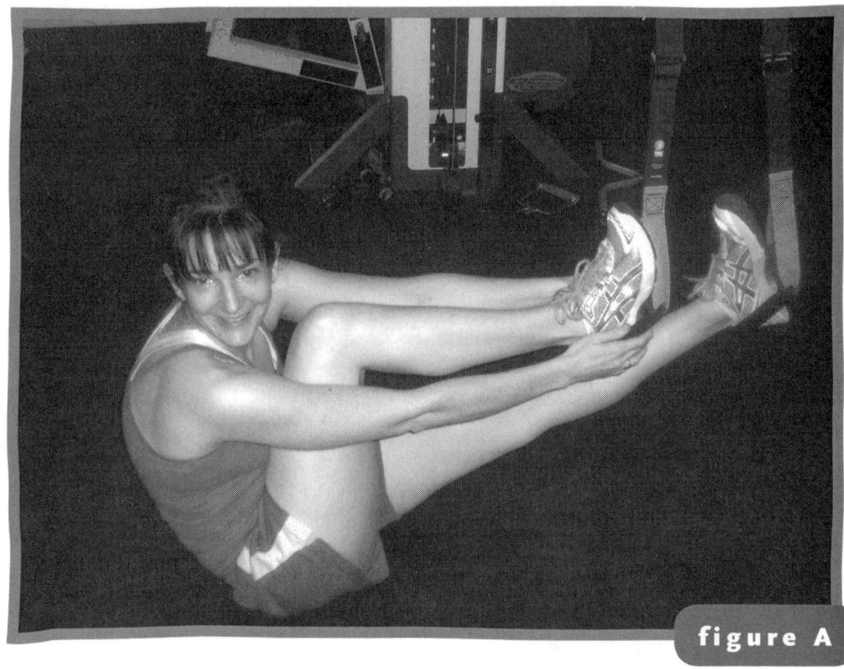

figure A

machine right smack dab in the middle of the weight floor, in our case—and hook the carabiner through the strap. But getting the handles to be the same height required some serious gymnastics. Every time we'd put our weight on one strap, the other would snap up to the ceiling, dropping us like a rock on the dirty gym floor.

Gym Buddy Allison demonstrates the peril involved with trying to get the two handles equal (see figure B).

The first two exercises we attempted were basic squats and lunges while holding onto the handles. We managed those with no undue stress. But exercise number three was a doozy. Designed to work the hamstrings and hip adductors, you start like this (see figure C).

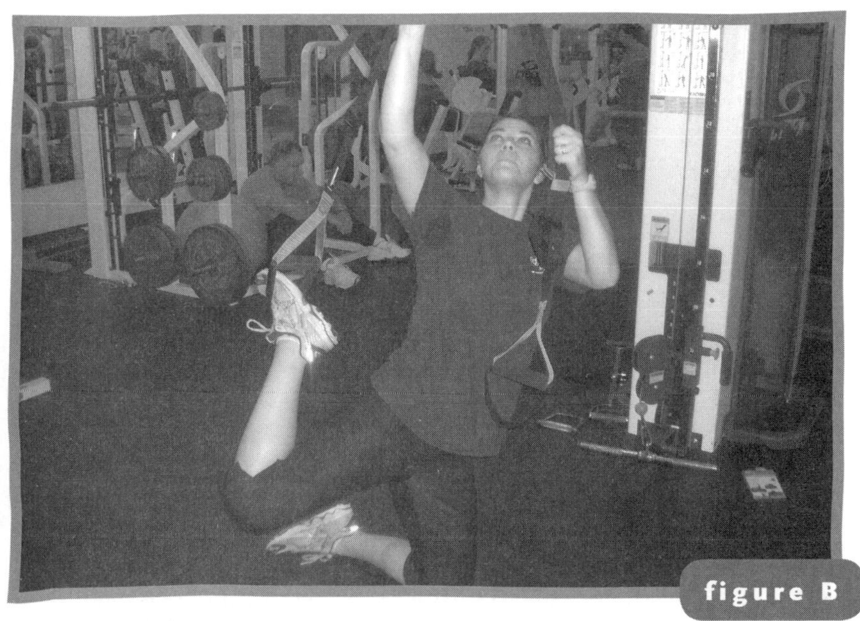

figure B

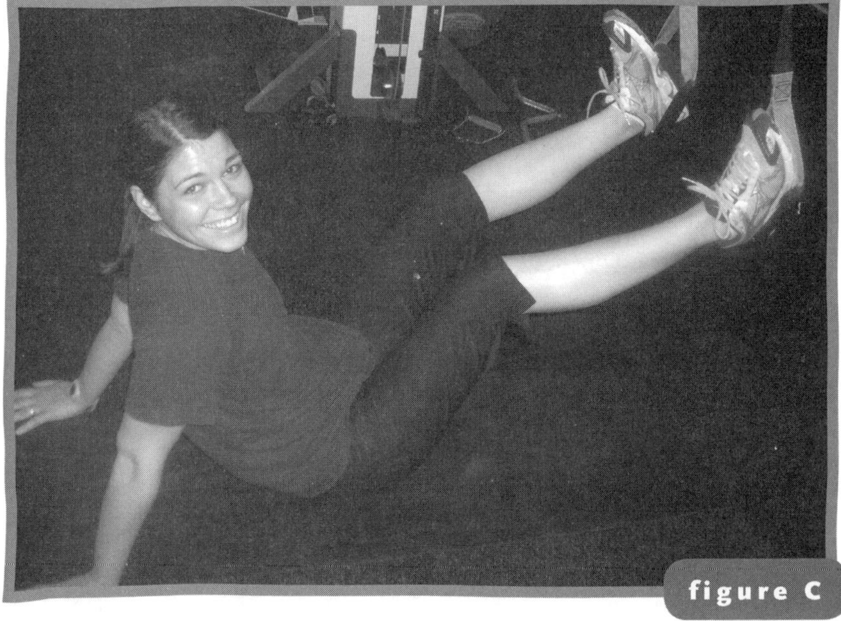

figure C

(As I took the picture, Allison actually said, "I'm ready for my exam now." I almost dropped the camera.)

And end like this (forcing the question: Which is the lesser evil—facing the wall o' mirrors or the track? See figure D).

Next up were push-ups. Not only were these an excellent burn—you just move your feet farther back until it is as difficult as you need—but they also encouraged several bystanders to give suspension training a try (see figure E).

(Not that anyone cares, but that little vein on each shoulder? I worked really, really hard for those vascular badges of honor. And I named them.)

Allison managed to make the push-up look a little less like falling and a lot more like fun. Which it was, if I do say so myself (see figure F).

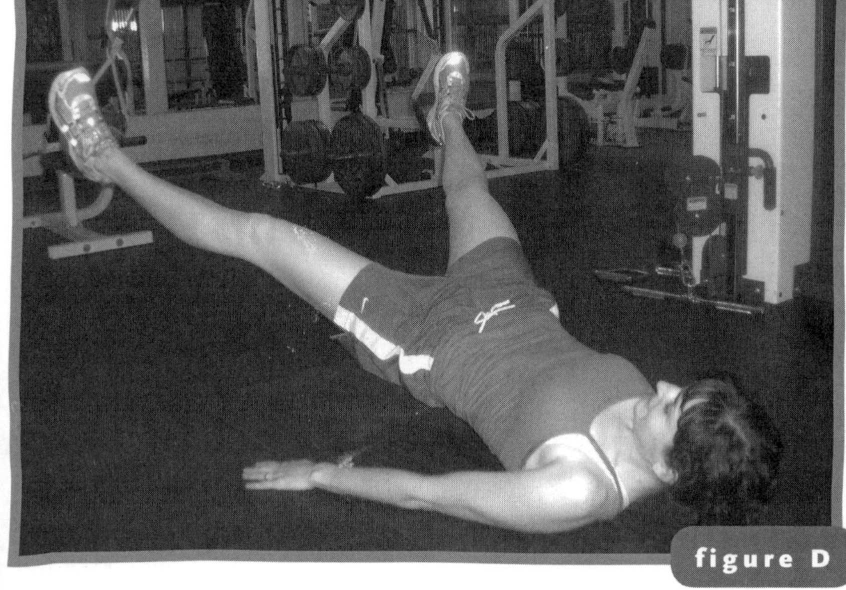

figure D

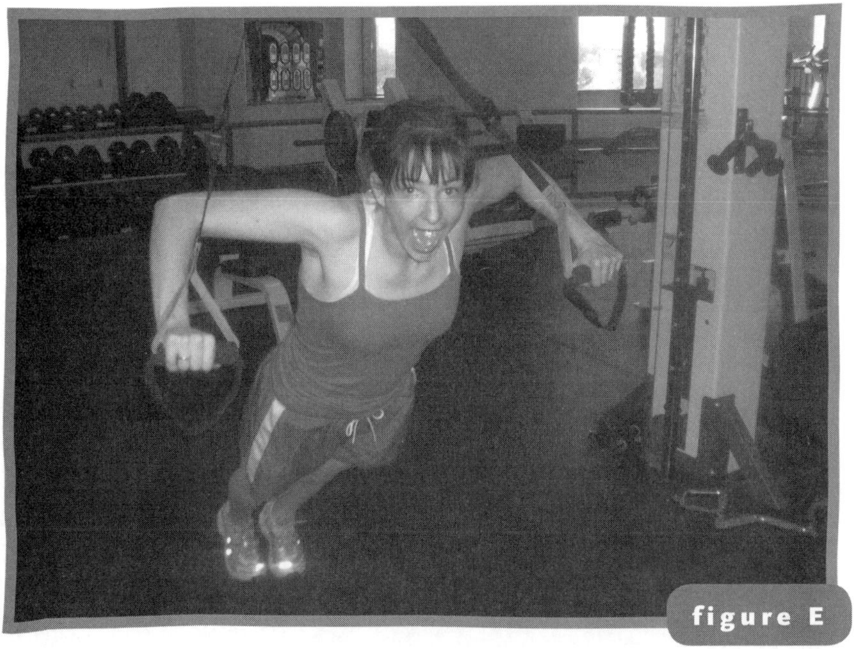

figure E

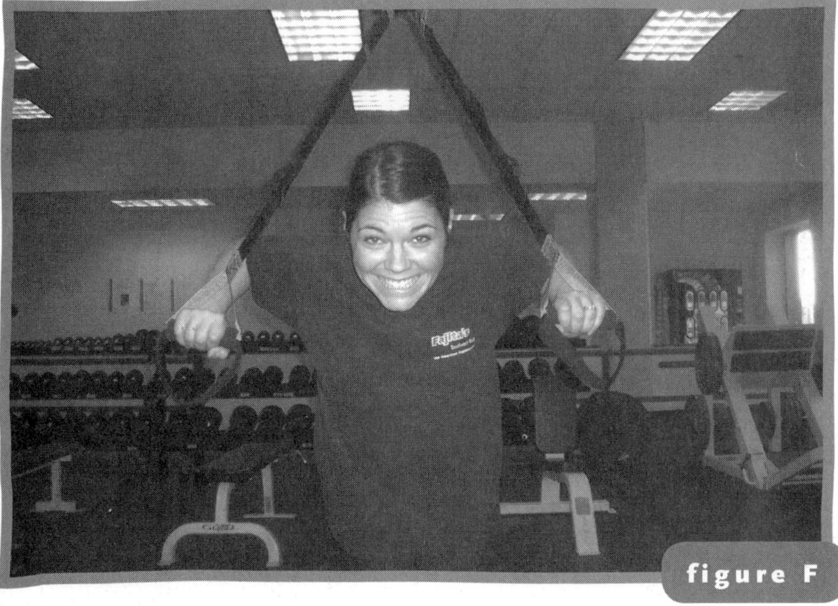

figure F

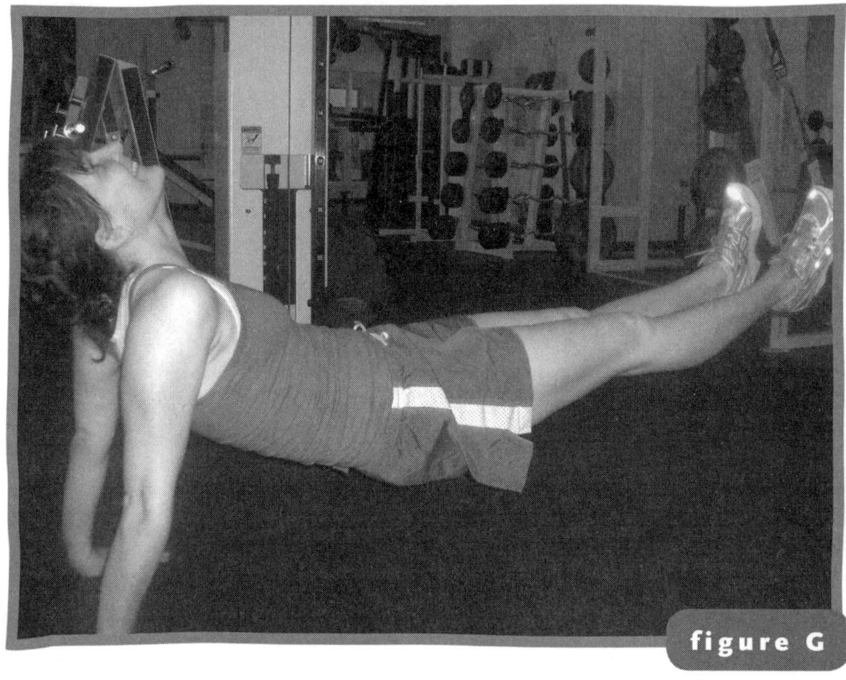

figure G

The coup d'état of the workout though was a move named the "supine pull-through." It should have been called Pure Ab Evil. Oh, sure, it looked easy enough on the Web site. This is how you start out (sort of) (see figure G).

Random Stranger: *You're doing it wrong.*

Me: *Unnhhhhh . . . ?*

RS: *In the picture (points to my handy dandy laminated workout card) her butt is higher than her feet. You're sagging.*

Me: *Huuummmmmmmhhhhh!*

RS: *It looks easy in the picture.*

Me: *Well, it's not! I can't lift my hips any higher or my legs fly apart!*

RS: *Oh, yeah! Like that stirrups move you were doing earlier? That was a good one. You should definitely do that one again.*

ME: *Ewwwwww....*

And this is . . . well, it's not at all how you are supposed to end but was as close as we could get. Yeah, Allison's butt's off the floor. And it's NOT easy, okay? It's ridiculously hard. That's right, punks (see figure H).

By this time we had gathered quite a crowd and so we challenged our friend (not to be confused with Random Stranger, above) to give it his best shot. Yep, not even a super-buff kickboxer guy could do it. (Although he did get really close. And managed to make it look better than either Allison or I did.) Plus, I had to show proof that Male Gym Buddies do exist! (see figure I).

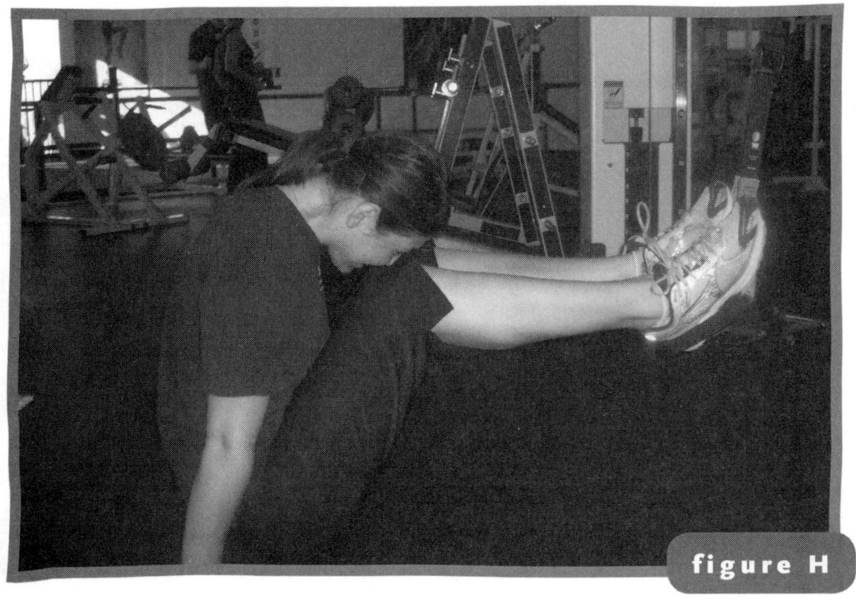

figure H

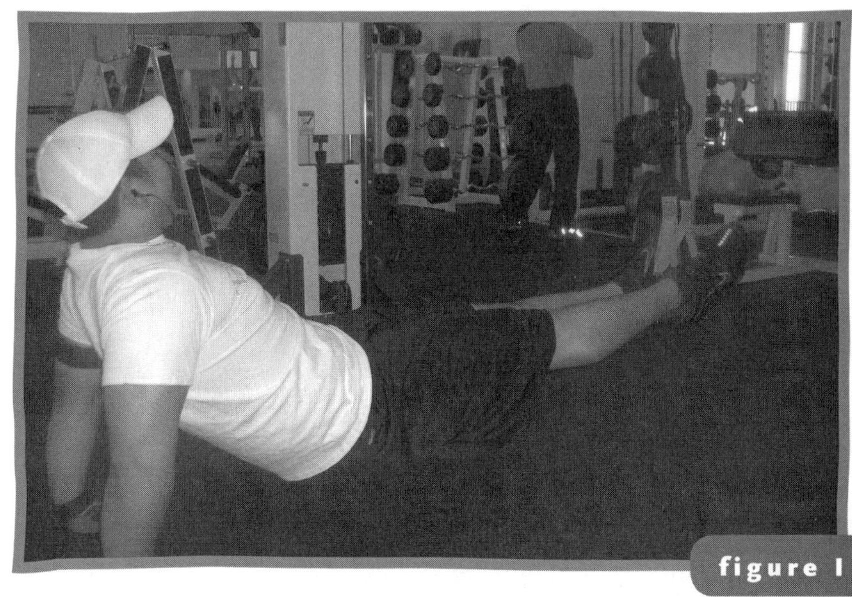

figure I

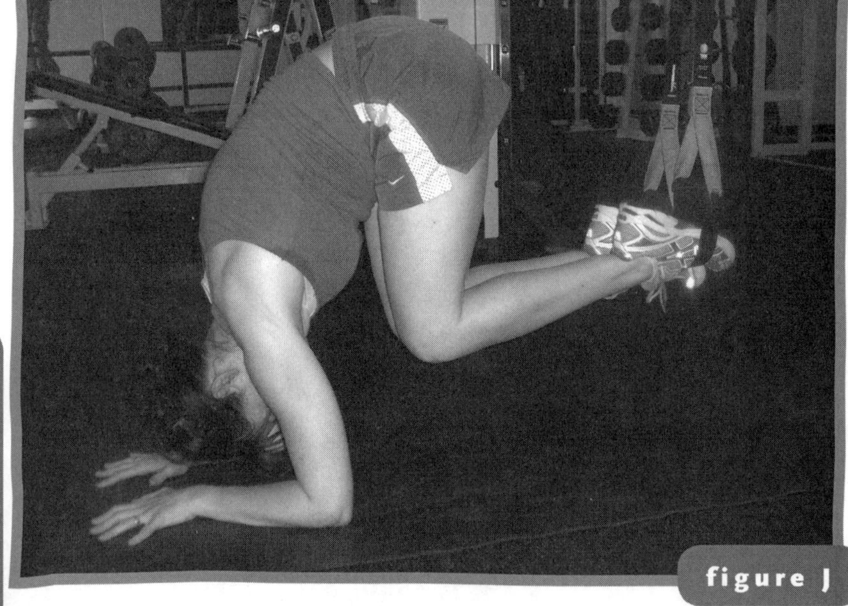

figure J

The final humiliation of the morning involved an ab crunch that, while easy enough to execute, ended in this fun-for-everyone pose (see figure J).

We concluded by using the suspension trainer to do some Pilates-type moves and stretch out our sore legs. Excitingly, this ended up being closer to aerial dancing than I ever could have dreamed! Both Gym Buddy Allison and I "took flight" and sailed gracefully (cough, cough) in circles around the floor (see figure K).

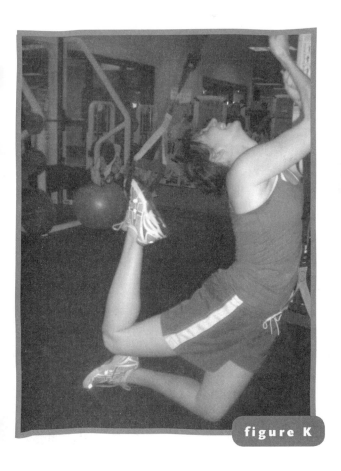

figure K

The best part of the day was after we finished our workout/giggle-fest, packed up all our gear, and apologized to everyone we irritated, we passed an open studio on our way down the stairs. Want to know what was inside it, hanging calmly from a ceiling beam far, far away from prying eyes? A brand spanking new TRX. That's right, after all the drama with stealing the chin-up bar and ticking off the regulars and basically taking over the weight floor, it turns out the Y already had one! It's like rain on your wedding day. It's a free ride when you've already paid. It's the good advice that you just didn't take. It's 10,000 spoons when all you need is a knife! Yes, it's *ironic,* dontcha think? (And now you're singing Alanis Morissette. You're welcome!)

Out of the Gym

UNFORTUNATELY, THIS EXPERIMENT had the dubious distinction of getting us kicked out of the gym. Or at least off part of the fitness floor. For a long time the personal trainers had been annoyed by our antics. Indeed, one male personal trainer parroting the oft-told axiom that men find strong women frightening, said of Gym Buddy Allison and me: "Those girls scare me."

My first reaction was, "Us? Scary??" We're about as scary as the Hamburgler. (Seriously, Ronald McDonald is scary. But if you met the Hamburgler in a dark alley, you know it'd start with "Gimme your wallet" and end with fist bumps and "Just messin' with you, man!") Perhaps the trainer was afraid that we'd do something stupid and make quadriplegics out of ourselves and sue the

Y. But I'm pretty sure that all-encompassing liability waiver we signed when we got our memberships prevents us from ever living that dream. Besides, while we try lots of different things, we don't do anything terribly risky. The worst we're in danger of are some wicked bruises, a rolled ankle, or possibly a pulled ab muscle from laughing too hard.

My second reaction was to puff out my chest and growl, "He *should* be scared, by golly! We could kick his butt!" And then I realized that anyone who says "by golly"—even in their imagination—is inherently not scary. Plus, I like to talk big (and kiss my biceps when no one's looking), but I really have no idea how to handle myself in a fight. In a showdown, I'm sure I'd be the one eating mat (see the Karate Experiment, chapter 12, for further proof). Allison and I can't even play basketball without apologizing every two minutes and saying, "No, really, you take another shot—I had the ball last time!"

Gym Buddy Mike has his own theory. "It's because you guys have no fear, and that's what personal trainers usually do—help people overcome their fears. He knows you don't need him." He added, "Take it as a compliment, really." It's true. I do not worship the personal trainers as the purveyors of all fitness knowledge. Which isn't to say that he is stupid. I'm sure he knows many things that I do not. I'm just saying that we dare to use the "weird" equipment and try out new exercises, and we're not reliant on the personal trainers to show us how.

Or perhaps he finds us scary because we are markedly unfeminine in the gym. Despite always wearing sports bras and pony tails, we routinely invade the male-dominated areas of the gym.

We wear weight gloves and talk about one-rep maxes. We can list seven different exercises to hit all three heads of your shoulder. We do CrossFit and pull-ups and handstand pushups. I even belched today—loudly—for good measure. We're working up to scratching ourselves.

I have to say I'm a little sad that he finds us "scary," for whatever reason, because ultimately I'd rather work with people and share knowledge than be fighting them for gym space. In the end, though, I'd rather be scary than weak, so if being strong makes me scary then bring it on.

In addition to the disdain of the personal trainers, this month also earned us a first in Gym Buddy History: our own personal warning sign! After working out for several weeks on the TRX, using both my own and the identical one that the Y has, the Gym Buddies and I were greeted one morning by a sign on the studio door (a studio open to the gym public, I might add) that read:

> "Equipment in this room is for use only with a personal trainer after the proper training.
>
> *Sincerely, Gym Management*"

It might as well have said:

> "Dear Charlotte, we fear you and think your crazy antics will land us in a law suit. If we knew a better way to get you kicked out of the gym, we'd do it, but in the meantime we're hoping that you don't see this sign so we can catch you doing something naughty (like exercising!) and give you the boot.
>
> *Sincerely, Gym Managment*"

I didn't do it but I was sorely tempted to tack on a Post-it note replying:

> "Dear YMCA, I would like to say that the TRX is probably the least risky piece of equipment in the gym. You could do more damage to life, limb, and property with an improperly wielded fifty-pound dumbbell than a couple of straps with handles on them. If you want to get worked up about something, how about cracking down on folks who sit on the locker room benches starkers? Now that's a health risk.
>
> *Sincerely, The Gym Buddies*"

The Results

NOW THAT I'VE LEFT YOU WITH THE IMAGE of nude eighty-year-olds lounging on benches burned into your retinas, let's discuss how suspension training fared as an actual workout. Since this Experiment replaced only our weight lifting (we kept our cardio the same), I didn't expect a huge change in body composition, and I was correct. My weight, body fat percentage, and measurements all stayed the same.

What I Liked

Where suspension training really shone was in its adaptability, portability, and flexibility. Quite honestly, if I were interested in setting up a home gym—which I'm not because then who would leave me passive-aggressive signage to brighten my day?—this would be the first piece of equipment I'd buy. Yes, even before a set of kettlebells (see chapter 9). Since suspension training uses only your own body weight and gravity as resistance, it is very light and therefore super portable. You can work every muscle group to failure with just a couple of nylon straps. I love the simplicity. In addition to being able to shove it into a carry-on, it is very easy to set up, adjust, and take down, whether it be in your hotel room, spare bedroom, or even outside attached to a telephone pole. This was one of the lowest-maintenance workouts I've ever tried.

Not only is it good for traditional-type strength training, it is also great for stretching and some Pilates moves. Pretty much every move engages your core because of the instability created by the straps. I've never been so sore in my torso, and I think I've got a pretty strong core.

And in regards to the age-old question of "Is bodyweight training enough?" I would have to say that you can get just as an effective workout using just your body and gravity as you can with iron.

What I Didn't Like

The main issue I have with suspension training is you are somewhat limited in the moves you can do. I suppose some of you are more imaginative than I am, but I tried every single exercise that came on the DVDs or the Web site, and there were a few body parts that left me stymied as to alternate exercises. After we were banned (for our own safety, I'm sure) from using the second TRX, the Gym Buddies and I moved out to the weight floor where we incorporated the TRX with some barbell and floor work to make a circuit that all of us enjoyed very much. So if you have the option, using the TRX with other forms of exercise equipment is the best of both worlds. But, really, that's not much of a downside.

It's spendy. The basic TRX package starts at $149.95. Or, if you are good with macramé, you can make your own, but that seems like a lot of effort.

Best Moment

The Gym Buddies and I quickly discovered that if we put a mat under our feet and backed waaay up, holding onto the handles of the TRX, we could then launch ourselves across the floor like some kind of dry-land wakeboarding. It was even still fun when Allison fell so hard she bruised her butt, and I got so tangled up in the ropes that it took two Gym Buddies to get me down. Sadly we were caught by Gym Management, who was not impressed with our party tricks. We were threatened with disciplinary action. I still say it was totally worth it.

P·E·R·S·O·N·A·L·|·E·S·S·A·Y

Fallible: On Making Mistakes in Public

During all my years of teaching, I've seen a lot. In a single quarter I had a student vomit, another have a stroke, and a third show up for the final with no teeth claiming police brutality. I was teaching as the Twin Towers fell and watched the chaos ensue via the Internet. I've even been mooned by an irate teenager who was upset that I wouldn't let him take the quiz he missed by showing up late. But the image that sticks with me the most from my professorial days was of a mistake. A huge mistake.

It was my first year teaching, and I made up for my nerves with bravado and humor. The class was one of those freshman behemoths required for every major, the kind of filter class that students hate taking and teachers hate teaching. Four days a week, I lectured from a podium in front of a huge screen dropped from the ceiling. The set-up was all modern and technical so whatever I had on my computer screen displayed on the screen. And thus my downfall began.

I had the habit of breaking up the class with humorous video clips I found on the Internet. I was not supposed to do this. In fact, I was strictly instructed to stick to the manual and its set of boring exercises. But like I said, I was nervous and eager to be liked and very, very young, so I did it anyhow. Until one day I mistyped the URL of the site I was looking for. I meant to have a funny site show up but instead landed on a hard-core porn site, complete with all the naughty pop-up windows that those sites spawn.

There was an audible gasp in the audience, and in the seconds it took for the mistake to travel to my brain, my body decided to act. Causing human resource directors everywhere to shudder in horror, I threw myself in front of the screen trying to block the image with my body. Unfortunately, as I'm sure you can imagine, this does not work with a projector and a screen of megaplex proportions. Instead, it looked as if I had thrown myself into the middle of a terribly lewd act. And for good measure, a very disturbing phrase was scrolling across the bottom of the screen—right across my stomach.

The students, being college kids, were wildly entertained until I managed to turn the projector off, and it might have ended there. Except that somehow word got back to the dean, and I was called in for an interview. And here's where it gets particularly cringe worthy. After having to describe in detail what exactly the picture was showing on the site to a man old enough to be my grandfather, I had to explain to him how it happened. Instead of simply admitting my mistake and asking for forgiveness, I tried to snow him. I babbled on about black widow sites and viruses and domain name hijacking and rerouting and any other technical details I could think of until at last I ran out of steam.

Sitting back and staring at me thoughtfully, he eventually said quietly, "They'll never hate you for making mistakes. Everyone does that. But they'll never respect you if you can't admit to those mistakes." I was too stunned to speak.

That is a lesson I took to heart. In every class I taught after that point, I would tell the students right at the beginning that I wasn't perfect and that most likely there was someone present who knew more than I did. (Which really came in handy the day I started a computer on fire. Seriously.) That they should tell me when I am wrong and accept when I did the same for them. That nobody should be afraid of making mistakes; the only important thing was to try.

It is a lesson that translates well to health and fitness. I see a lot of people avoiding healthy activities out of fear of making mistakes. If you exercise in a gym setting, then that fear is multiplied by the very public nature of the environment. For instance, a few months back I saw a woman pick up a resistance band. After glancing around a few times, she finally stepped on it and pulled up on the handles, just like she'd seen a personal trainer do with a client. Unfortunately, she didn't have a good lock on the band, and it whipped out from under her feet and smacked her across the face. I had to fake a coughing fit for a good five minutes to keep from laughing until I fell off my treadmill, it was that funny. It was certainly embarrassing. So what did the woman do? Dropping the handles, she stepped over the band and walked away as if nothing had happened. But her beet-red face betrayed her. I wanted to run after her and tell her that it's okay—I've totally snapped myself with the resistance band too—and then show her how to put it under the groove in your shoe so it can't come loose. But she was gone, hopefully not to hide under a rock. If she had stuck around long enough, I would have told her how I actually put a hole in my super-tight spandex pants when I snapped myself on the butt with a jump rope while trying to show off during boot camp.

Making mistakes is not about being dumb, it's about being teachable. It's about admitting that I don't have all the answers and that I have a lot to learn from other people. I've learned that I will never be perfect at anything the first time I try it. Chances are I'll never be perfect at it, period. I've also learned that nobody likes a perfect person anyhow. People are drawn to those who can make mistakes and learn from them. Our fallibility, it's a gift.

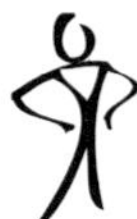

september

chapter nine

September
Kettlebells

I'M GOING TO TELL YOU right up front: The best thing about kettlebells is all the inappropriate jokes they inspire. Not to knock them as a fitness tool—they give a seriously hard-core workout—but the humor they provide is priceless. It may be the only time you get to look your Gym Buddy in the eye and say "Hey, niiice rack!" and not get slapped.

The Theory

ONCE, THE ONLY CHOICE THAT EARLY TWENTIETH-CENTURY Russian weight lifters had (funny how one man's deprivation becomes another man's inspiration), these iron cannonballs with attached handle—think twee little purse but with a skull shoved inside it—have become the newest fitness sensation overnight. These days you'll find them in nearly every gym, in dedicated kettlebell classes, and on a plethora of fitness DVDs. Not to mention they have their own YouTube channel, which is pretty much the gold standard of cool in this decade. The reason for their celeb status is that they boast a combined cardio and strength workout, all-in-one fat-torching thirty-minute circuit. But if you hang around the fitness world long enough, you learn that people often get all breathless over the newest gadget or technique only to find out six months down the road that not only does it not work, but it probably causes cancer to boot. So I had to know: Is this just another fitness gadget fad destined to gather dust between your BOSU ball and your ab roller, or is it really the life-changing workout they say it is?

My first kettlebell was a little red fifteen-pounder so adorable that I immediately christened her Tinkerbell. (As if you don't name your fitness equipment!) I quickly discovered, however, that that might have been a misnomer. Popping in the instructional DVD that came in the box, I started with the most basic move: the swing. Standing with your feet wider than your hips, you swing the 'bell from between your legs, arcing it in front of you and then up just past shoulder height. The move is designed to get your heart pumping and also work a variety of muscles from your quads to your back and on up to your shoulders. Just as I was settling in to a nice rhythm, focusing on "driving with my butt" and thinking how entertaining all this hip thrusting was going to be on the weight floor, Tinkerbell struck. My knee, to be precise, thudding loudly into my kneecap on the bottom end of the swing. I saw stars and then bit my tongue as I collapsed on the floor. It was a warning: No matter how candy colored, the kettlebell will be taken seriously.

The Workout

Rule #1: You must pay attention.

The next day at the gym, with a bruise that allowed me to work the phrase "mafia hit" into every conversation, I sternly instructed the Gym Buddies on this lesson. And lest we forgot it, by the end of our first kettlebell workout, no less than five people had stopped to tell us to "be careful with that thing; don't throw it through the mirrors!" You will be happy to know that no mirrors—or kneecaps—were broken in the making of this Experiment. Egos? Well, that's another story.

Rule #2: Pick a good workout.

As with any new fitness trend, there are a handful of people that really know what they're doing, and then there are the rest of us. This wasn't so bad when the fitness tool du jour was resistance bands (worst case scenario: wicked welts in unseemly places) but hand a bunch of untrained fitness nuts a loaded ball-o-iron and you're just asking for trouble. The problem is it's hard to find an "expert" when the thing has really only been around for a couple of years. Besides, I'm cheap. Why pay someone when the Internet will tutor me for free?

The first workout I picked was a middle-of-the-road version from a popular women's fitness magazine. Lady mags are safe right? I should have known that something was up when all the pictures used to illustrate the "Kettlebell Workout" article had the model using *dumbbells*. After an hour of the Gym Buddies asking me, "How is this different?" I realized I was going to have to dig deeper.

So then I went to the source—a Russian body building Web site that boasted moves like—and I am not kidding you—the one-finger pull-up. In the warm-up. Go big or go home, right? Let's just say that any workout that ends with old ladies running across the gym to my aid screaming, "Oh, my dear, are you okay?!?!?" is my kind of workout.

Rule #3: Form is everything.

It was the renegade rows that did me in. Also called floor rows or plank rows, the move has you hold a plank, but instead of putting your hands on the floor, you balance on two weights. You then do a "row" by lifting one weight at a time up to your armpit while still holding the plank. A killer move, they've long been a staple in my iron repertoire, so I did not anticipate the kettlebells throwing me like they did. One minute I was perched on top of two twenty-five-pound 'bells o' wonder; the next I was nose to the ground in a heap of floor-burned spandex (oh, right, it's called "wicking fabric" these days). And it wasn't that it is a hard lift, per se, but rather the gym equivalent of that circus trick where the elephant balances on the beach ball. One little wobble in my wrist and the pachyderm went wild like Dumbo's mama. I ended up with rubber grit in my teeth and a chorus of laughing Gym Buddies. The little old ladies were not amused.

Floor burns and ego burns notwithstanding, the workout kicked my butt. The next day I was sore in places I didn't even know had muscles. As the Gym Buddies and I worked through the month, we discovered that just like with traditional weight lifting, form is everything. One of the comments we got most frequently from curious onlookers—and there were a lot of those for this Experiment—was: "You guys are going to kill your backs!" It is true that with traditional weight lifting, the rule is "Never swing the weights." (This rule is second only to "Never drop the weights"—especially true in our gym where they put the weight floor right over the childcare. There have been reports of pants wetting. And that was just the staff.) Properly using the kettlebells requires a lot of swinging. Swinging that, if you're not careful to use your legs, butt, and hips to generate the momentum, really will throw your back out. The Gym Buddies and I learned the hard way that it is well worth your time and money to find a certified instructor to teach you the basics. After a couple of classes, we were good to go.

Rule #4: Go heavy.

Because you get to swing the weights, and many moves allow you to use two hands to control the 'bells, you can handle a lot more weight than you are used to. To get the full effect of this workout—*after* you've made sure your form is stellar, of course—pick up a seriously heavy weight.

After a week of not seeing results with Tinkerbell, the Gym Buddies and I borrowed a twenty-five-pound 'bell we called "Sheila" and some forty-five-pounders we named "The Berthas." Once we got comfortable with the moves and our form, we used Sheila and The Berthas almost exclusively. I know they market those teeny little fifteen- and ten-pounders very aggressively to women, but they are really only good for working small muscles. To get the full effect of the workout, you really need to go heavier. Don't worry, little girl, we won't hurt you. Much.

Rule #5: Keep it short.

Kettlebell workouts are intense. If you can talk through it, you're not doing it properly. And, also, if you're chatting, you're going to conk yourself in the kneecap. Ahem. Because of the high intensity of the workout, you can keep it under thirty minutes and still get a great cardio and strength workout. It's short but plan on working hard. Like puking hard.

Rule #6: Wear wristbands.

Oh, yes, I'm talking about those terry cloth staples that used to only be cool in the '80s or at Wimbledon but now, thanks to hip-hop, are making a major comeback. Except that just like with anything you see in a hip-hop video, you can't wear it like they do—high up on one arm. (Note: This rule also applies to sparkly pasties, excessively baggy pants, and untied shoes, yo!) You will actually want those bands pulled down over your tender wrist bones. Also, take off your watch, rings, and any bracelets. Make sure to put them in a safe place, or you'll end up sans expensive Bulgari watch like Gym Buddy Megan.

The thing that nobody mentions about kettlebells is the wrist thumpage. Every time you swing that sucker back up and "rack" it on your forearm, you are basically hitting yourself with a twenty-five-pound weight. It hurts. Bad. Sometimes they tell you to rack the weight on your shoulder or bicep. I'm telling you that it hurts to hit yourself *anywhere* with a twenty-five-pound weight. Just don't forget to take the wristbands off when you are done, or everyone will think you're a cutter, and next thing you know, you're on reality TV having an intervention. Nobody wants that.

In the Gym

AFTER AT LEAST 200 PEOPLE WROTE ME on my blog to tell me that the key to curing wrist thumpage and to getting a better burn is to go to a trained instructor, I finally broke down and signed the Gym Buddies and me up for a lesson. Sadly, it was only to be one lesson, as the first lesson was free and everything after that cost more money than a mother of four children whose favorite foods are artichokes and steamed crab legs—but hey, at least they like healthy stuff, right?—would want to spend. So I was determined to get as much out of our one class as possible. Translation: I was going to be really obnoxious and ask way too many questions.

Our lesson started off well with Gym Buddy Allison and I forgetting that I had signed us up for the class. Thankfully, Gym

Buddy Krista was on the ball and reminded us by shooting emphatic looks at us through the studio windows until we clued in. We made it in at the last second. Warm-ups were light floor aerobics, entertaining mostly because Allison forgot she wasn't in our Hip-Hop Hustle class and did a very cool dip in the middle of her grapevine left. Well, it would've looked cool if she weren't the only one dipping. And if we'd had Turbo Jennie's disco ball going. As it was, we just giggled a lot.

The class itself was a thirty-minute butt-kicker. I already knew the power of kettlebells to get the heart rate pumping, but it was even better having someone else kick my butt rather than me yelling random instructions at the Gym Buddies. I completely pitted out my shirt in the first ten minutes—the sign of a really great workout. The rest was just sweaty gravy. In addition to the kettlebell swings, lunges, and presses that we were used to, we got to try out a few new moves. My favorite was the one where you hold the handle and rotate the 'bell around your head. I believe the move was called an "around the world," and not only was it a great shoulder burn, but it was also good for my ego. (My head being the world. Get it?) My only complaint with the class was that even after much pestering from me, the instructors didn't do much to teach proper kettlebell form, resulting in one Gym Buddy with bad back pain, a common first-time kettlebell complaint, and exactly what we were trying to prevent. In a strange bit of fitness guerilla warfare, the teacher explained to me afterwards that in the paid classes, emphasizing and correcting proper form would be a priority. Apparently you get what you pay for.

The Results

I WAS CERTAIN THAT AFTER ONE MONTH of doing these killer kettlebell circuits three times a week that the Gym Buddies and I were going to see big results. But some Experiments just don't work out how I think they will. Just as in life, some things just don't make sense. Take, for instance, The New Kids On The Block much-hyped comeback song "Summertime." I mean the girl in the song is walking the beach in "flip flops, half shirt, short shorts, miniskirt." Who wears short shorts *and* a miniskirt? Was it a skort? If so, why didn't one of the Joeys just sing "skort"? Granted, skorts are generally for preschoolers who can't be trusted to keep their panties covered (Hush, Madonna, I said *preschoolers),* but do singers not actually think about their lyrics before they sing them? Also, NKOTB, I realize you've been out of the boy-band loop for a couple of decades but a) half shirts are not cool anymore, and b) nobody calls them half shirts anymore. Seriously, every time I listen to that song, I get dumber. And yet it's still on my playlist. Stupid catchy beat.

What I Liked

1. KETTLEBELLS ARE VERY VERSATILE. You can use them to do traditional lifts, or you can swing them to get your cardiovascular system involved. At first I couldn't really see a benefit to using them over the dumbbells, but as the month went on, I began to see that they really do offer a different element to your workout. Especially once I figured out proper swinging form. They even change up more static moves like the Turkish Get-Up by adding an element of instability.

2. THERE'S A LOT OF BANG FOR YOUR BUCK THERE. If I were investing in a home gym, these babies would be one of the first things I'd buy. I'd get a set of fifteens, twenty-fives, and fifties. It's easy to make a tight little weight/cardio circuit with just a few kettlebells.

3. THEY ARE EASIER TO GRIP THAN A TRADITIONAL DUMBBELL. I loved them for doing things like the farmer's carry and lunges, while Gym Buddy Allison adored the windmill.

4. THE COOL FACTOR. First off, they're just cute—like wee purses. That could take a man's head off. Second, everyone at the gym wanted to see them. Not only did everybody stop to watch—frankly, not an unusual occurrence for me—but they were all really interested in trying them. Third, they inspire all kinds of cute names. One trainer kept asking me how my "cowbells" were going. "Kettleball" was also a favorite.

What I Didn't Like

1. THE WRIST THUNK. Like I mentioned before, wristbands help, but they don't stop the bruising. When I asked our free instructor about it, his only recommendation was to toughen up. As you get stronger, you can control the 'bell better but it still thumps.

2. THE STEEP LEARNING CURVE. This isn't particular to kettlebells, but there really is a technique needed, and it was hard to catch on from YouTube and the Internet alone, almighty sources of iffy knowledge though they are. A class or private instruction would be better, but you will probably have to pay for those unless your mooching skills are better than mine are (in which case, please write me and share your secrets!).

And here's where it gets weird. This month, I gained 2 percent body fat, all my measurements went up by at least half an inch, and—even though I pretend to be above caring about this, we all know the truth is that I do—I gained three pounds. For how hard I worked, I was very surprised by this. Under normal circumstances,

Best Moment

By far the best moments in this workout were all the times I got to yell across a crowded weight floor, "Thrust with your hips! Come on, guys, really clench your butt and drive that pelvis forward!" as we all stood in a line in front of the mirror like so many randy frat boys. I told you this Experiment was inappropriate!

these kinds of results would make me inclined to write off kettlebells as a fad. But I think, honestly, the failure this time around was with me and not the workout. There were hormones involved. Not to mention a great deal of outside stress. In the end, it was a very quick, adaptable, and efficient workout. I would totally recommend it. Just watch your kneecaps.

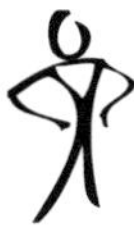

P·E·R·S·O·N·A·L·|·E·S·S·A·Y

Stopping the Stomach Wars: Making Peace with Your Tummy

My friend Liz and I have been best friends since elementary school. We thought we were two halves of the same person and campaigned relentlessly to our parents to never, ever separate us. After all, a multitude of friendship bracelets, twin My Child dolls, and even an actual padlock hooking us together couldn't be wrong!

As we grew up though, life and husbands took us to opposite ends of the country, and we became Christmas-card and the occasional e-mail buddies. Recently we have re-bonded over —get this—skin. See, in addition to sharing a love of running, we also birthed several human beings and have the marks to prove it.

Back in our My Child (like Cabbage Patch dolls but creepier) days, we often fantasized about having twins and raising them next door to each other. But our fantasies were noticeably void of several truths: sex (This was pre-Jamie Lynn after all.); the work/home balance (We were planning on joining the circus. Apparently all those babies were cared for by clowns. Not a bad gig, now that I think about it.); and, of course, the toll on our bodies.

Stress incontinence, stretch marks, wayward nips, and the ubiquitous "mummy tummy" were not part of the dream. Fifteen years later, I'd call them more of a nightmare.

There are a few lucky ladies who escape pregnancy and breastfeeding blemish free, but for most of us, being a mother definitely affects the way we work out. Gym Buddy Krista has a "two air jack maximum" in TurboKick before having to leave class to use the bathroom despite always going before class starts. A Gym Buddy from Seattle refers to her post-nursing chest as "rocks in socks" and, despite being an A cup, has to pour them into two sports bras to keep them from heading for the border. As for me, I have stretch marks from knee to clavicle. So much so that my oldest son christened me The Tiger Lady when he was three. It doesn't matter how good my abs are, the world will never see them in the light of day. Although you are welcome to admire my kneecaps as much as your little heart desires.

But it is the mummy tummy—or twin skin (a slight misnomer as I've only ever had very large singletons)—that has brought Liz and me together again. Last week she sent me an e-mail that is probably the number-one question women ask me. (You really don't want to know the number-one question men ask me. Of course, after reading this, they'll probably ask it a lot less.) Liz writes:

"I feel like no matter how many crunches I do or what technique I use, my belly just doesn't look that great. I have lost all my weight and even more, so I don't think that's it. Under the loose, wrinkly skin, I can feel the muscles and definition, but it doesn't show at all. Have you found a way around that (not involving a scalpel or paper cutter)? It's discouraging to work so hard but to not see any results. My belly is flat, but not really sexy. Just flat and saggy. Any thoughts?"

Paper cutter aside (Dear Liz, that was a horrible mental image), the short answer: Welcome to motherhood. Your stomach is simply one of many sacrifices you will make for your kids.

The slightly longer answer: Many (male) trainers have told me that the secret to this problem is to lose body fat. They all swear that the twin skin will tighten up on its own and that those sexy ab muscles will show once that pesky fat is gone. I have two problems with that answer: a) women need fat to live, and b) it just isn't true.

I hope I'm not going to regret this, but in the interest of helping women everywhere feel better about themselves, I'm going to give you a guided tour of my abs.

First things first: I generally avoid the use of any number when writing about working out, as numbers can be very triggering for people with eating disorders, and I have a significant number of readers that either have been or are disordered. So, if this kind of thing bothers you, please stop reading here. (I know, that's like a red sign pointing at the text below, but you know what you need, so please take gentle care of yourself.)

My body fat percentage in these pictures is 13.8 percent (I had my body fat tested hydrostatically, in the dunk tank, so this number is very accurate.) This is very low for a woman (average is 30 percent, most women aim for 20–25 percent). Doctors usually say that women need at least 10 percent just to survive and about 14 percent to menstruate. A popular workout guru whom I contacted through their Web site assured me that anything below 18 percent would give me "flat abs," and that below 16 percent, I'd have visible ab definition all the way down.

As you can see, that just isn't true. Now, don't get me wrong, I'm *not* complaining. My stomach looks flat in fitted clothing; I can wear a (one-piece) suit with only minor embarrassment; and I do have some visible ab musculature. However, there is obviously a lot of damage. A is pointing at some visible scars from random surgeries I've had (no expendable organs left here!). B and F show that my top two abs are visible (they would have been more prominent if I'd taken the pic in better lighting after my morning workout, but I'm lazy so this is post beans-for-dinner.) C shows stretch mark central. And D shows the line where I normally ride my pants thereby avoiding the, ahem, overhang you see in the picture. In addition to the excess skin on the sides, you can also see the loose skin in the little hood over my belly button (see figure L).

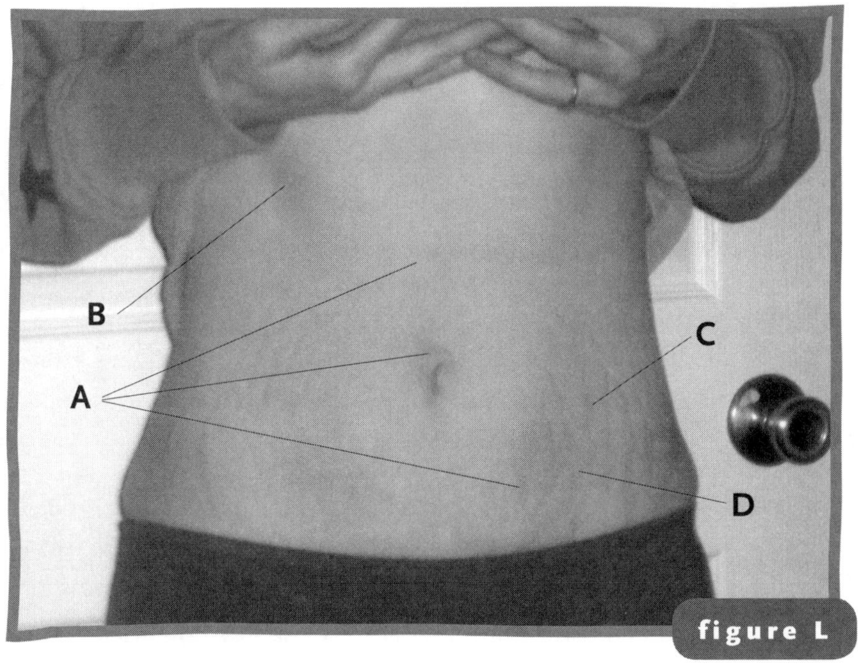

figure L

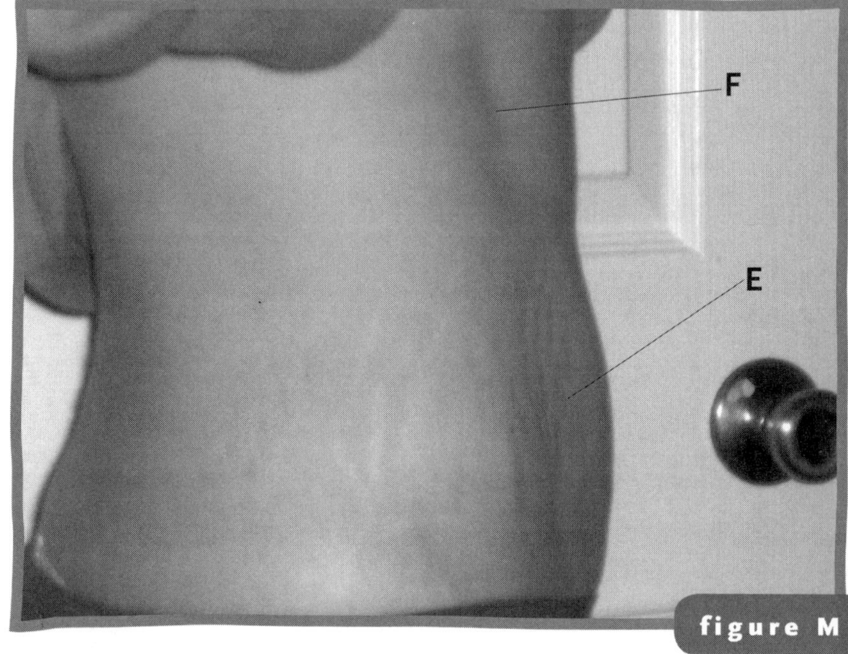

figure M

This is the money shot. Just because I love you all so much and wanted to be completely honest, I did not suck it in (see E). For those of you that are into numbers, I "pinch" at 3mms on my stomach with the calipers. I have *no extra fat to lose* (on my stomach, anyhow—thighs are a whole other story.) All of that you see is loose skin. Plain and simple, this is my stomach after having five kids (see figure M).

All of the beautiful sculpted abs you see on post-partum Trista Rehn, Jessica Alba, Nicole Richie, and the like? Genetics and Photoshop. Airbrushed tans and surgery. They are lucky and they are enhanced. Ladies, for most of us, this goal of perfectly flat abs is not only unrealistic but downright crazy making. A little below the belly bulge is *normal.* Gents (any of you that are still reading and haven't run from the room in horror yet), please manage your expectations. Your opinion means a lot to us. These are the tummies that carried your babies. Just love them.

Women, I truly hope that this helps you feel better about yourself. We have gestated and birthed babies. We have cuddled lovers. We have cradled the very old and nursed the very young. We are beautiful the way we are.

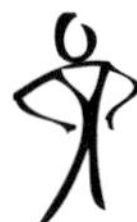

chapter ten

October

High Intensity Interval Training

IF FITNESS HAS A MAGIC BULLET, this is supposed to be it—and not just because the acronym reads like a directive. HIIT, or high intensity interval training, is the rare workout both beloved by fitness professionals and endorsed by researchers. What about the exerciser? Well, most of us love to hate it. There's puking involved.

It was the research study heard around the world. Well, my world anyhow. After studying social psychology in college, I fell in love with research when I got a job as a summer intern with the official position of tricking people. In case you've never had the privilege of being part of a study with human subjects, I'll just warn you now: the vast majority involve deception. Especially if they are paying you. My job that glorious summer was to tell people that we were doing a taste test of chocolate ice cream flavors and lead them into a cool room filled with bowls of ice cream where they got to eat to their heart's content and then fill out a survey about the flavors. After they were gone, I had the ignominious pleasure of weighing all their garbage to see how much of the pre-measured but unlimited servings of ice cream they had eaten. In short, I got to see how much people will eat when they think no one is watching them. This will not surprise you: they eat a lot. And scream a lot too. Especially when they find out you not only tricked them into betraying their gluttonous instincts but are then publishing a paper describing their gluttony. And for all this I got paid $4.25 an hour. Plus, of course, all the ice cream I could eat.

Ever since the Summer of Ice Cream (and Screaming), I will read anything with "research" or "study" or even "ice cream" in the title. I have been known to wet myself if the phrase "ethical review board" is uttered (that means humans were the subjects!). So when I came across a piece of fitness research that was not only conducted on human beings—as opposed to lab rats, monkeys, or reality show contestants (now there's a concept that should have gone before an ethical review board)—but also revolutionized how we thought about cardio, well all I'm going to say is there were beams from heaven and angelic singing involved. I had to try it.

The Theory

To test the efficacy of HIIT versus old-skool steady-state cardio, Dr. Steve Boucher, an Australian researcher from UNSW, took two groups of overweight women, assigning one group to the HIIT workout and the other to forty minutes of moderate-intensity work on a stationary bike. The first group performed twenty minutes broken into intervals of eight seconds maximal sprinting followed by twelve seconds of recovery. The second group just pedaled. For their sake, I'm hoping they at least got their own fan and access to Bravo because a *Project Runway* marathon would be the only thing that would make forty butt-searing minutes on a bike less horrible. At the end of the fifteen-week study, researchers measured weight lost and fat lost.

What did those wacky Aussies discover in their great bike race to nowhere? The HIIT group lost 2.5 kg (5.5 pounds) of fat, but when they took out the two subjects with a BMI of less than twenty (seriously, what were those two skinny chicks doing in the study in the first place?), the experimental group lost an astounding 4.5kg (9.9 pounds) of fat. And that's not talking total *weight* lost—although 9.9 pounds lost over fifteen weeks would be considered successful—but *fat* loss, which meant the subjects did the nearly impossible feat of keeping most of their lean muscle while ditching the jiggly stuff. As anyone who has tried to lose weight will tell you, losing fat while maintaining muscle is very difficult to do.

The control group on the other hand gained 0.5 Kg (1.1 pound) of fat. Another fact about research: being in the control group always sucks. (Unless you're testing medication, and then being in the control group means you get paid ridiculous amounts of money to eat sugar pills. Awesome!) The other shocker of the study was that in the HIIT group, a greater proportion of fat lost came from the hips, butt, and thighs. Can you think of anything more magical?

Lest you think this was one study performed on a small group of people, this research—and most research like it—was built on the foundation created by Nishimura Tabata, who first studied the use of HIIT to increase the performance of Olympic-caliber athletes. His intervals of twenty seconds work followed by ten seconds rest are more grueling than the ones used in the Australian study. Tabata and his colleagues achieved impressive results with his "Tabata Method," and the Australian study proved that those results don't just pertain to world class athletes.

The Workout

BEING EITHER CRAZY OR OVERLY OPTIMISTIC—you pick—I set up a program doing the HIIT intervals three times a week. For added fun, I roped in my long-suffering Gym Buddy Allison. What's the fun of pedaling until you puke if you don't have anyone to hold the bucket for you? For this first Experiment, we kept the intervals exactly the same as in the study, performing them on the bike for twenty minutes. Although we didn't realize until the end of the Experiment that I'd switched the work and rest periods, so for the month we stuck with twelve seconds of work followed by eight seconds of rest. For those of you bad at math—or just too tired to be bothered, like me—that's sixty intervals or twenty minutes. In between HIIT days, we lifted weights per our usual (uninspired) routine.

In later Experiments, we have incorporated HIIT in various forms of sprinting, rowing, squatting, and jump roping, including a particularly evil brand of interval on a treadmill called a Zoomer, which I will explain later. If you feel like trying these at home—and why wouldn't you? I haven't told you about the puke yet—note that if watching a clock is too difficult to do, there are "Tabata timers" that you can download for free off the internet. (Yep, there's an app for that!) Basically that means you are listening to a track on your iPod or phone that beeps at preprogrammed intervals. There is no music involved. Although it will keep your kids from stealing your iPod and has the added bonus of making you look crazy. Because the best parenting tactic I've found is to be unpredictable—nothing makes the little darlings behave like wondering if Mommy has lost her mind. And you thought you were just buying a fitness book!

In The Gym

MY FIRST ORDER OF BUSINESS in starting my very first Great Fitness Experiment was to misremember the research. Nothing says scientific rigor like "oops." But as you will quickly discover, my Experiments, while highly entertaining, are educational only insofar as you can put up with a great deal of academic fuzziness. This is how I found myself marching into the gym on the first day of October armed with nothing more than faulty knowledge and a best friend who, bless her heart, is always game for anything.

As we set up our bikes—not the fancy Spin kind mind you, but the large, clunky upright deals with plastic pedals and those huge seats that both lift and separate your butt cheeks (not an unpleasant feeling once you get used to it)—I explained to Gym Buddy Allison, "It's simple! All we do is sprint as hard as we can for twelve seconds and then pedal slowly for eight seconds. Repeat for twenty minutes and we're done!" I hadn't even started and already I had gotten the magic interval backwards.

"That's it?" she asked. See, in our fervor to "lose the baby weight"—her first, my fourth (you may commence gasping in either horror or awe now)—we'd been doing two hours of cardio every day.

"Yep! Not only is it shorter, but we'll burn more fat, and more of it will come from our saddlebags!"

"Okay," she shrugged and climbed on. "What resistance do I set it to?"

"Um . . . hard?" I didn't know. The study didn't say.

The study also didn't mention that after the first five minutes you see stars. Ten minutes into it, and the stars meld into a long tunnel with a light at the end. By fifteen minutes of this on-again-off-again torture, you can no longer see nor hear anything but the blinking red timer on your bike. By nineteen minutes you will be sure you will vomit and/or faint. Conveniently, at twenty minutes, you will fall off your bike.

As we lay in a puddle of our own bodily fluids between the orthopedic-shod feet of the contingent of concerned senior citizens that populate our YMCA, trying just to regain basic breathing and sensory functions, Allison growled, "I'd better wake up tomorrow with a six pack."

And that's the problem with HIIT that all of the research failed to mention: It hurts. *Bad.*

But I was determined to stick with it for thirty days. After all, there was so much to recommend it: According to the buckets of reliable research, it increases fat loss, endurance, oxygen utilization, post-exercise fat burning, and human growth hormone, just to name a few. Plus it decreases time spent exercising. Not to mention that every fitness guru, magazine, and show was singing the praises of interval training. Dare I say it? HIIT was the new spandex in the fitness world. So if the price of all that healthy goodness is a bit of pain, then bring it!

We stuck with our program. . . for the first week. Here's something else the fitness magazines never mention about interval training: It's really hard to motivate yourself to do it. It's hard enough to get your butt in the gym every day, but it becomes a Sisyphean task when you know your workout is going to involve stars, tunnel vision, and possible vomit. Even if it is only twenty minutes. What we ended up with was managing to get the bike intervals in about twice a week—for twenty minutes if both Allison and I made it to the gym to shame each other into it, but only ten-to-fifteen minutes if we were on our own. I tell you, I spent many a sweat drenched session wondering what on earth those researchers had done to motivate those formerly sedentary, overweight people to do this killer routine for fifteen weeks. Large sums of money must have been involved. Or threatening to make them read all the tabloid stories about Brad Pitt and Angelina Jolie. Perhaps both.

About halfway through our Experiment though, something strange started to happen. It didn't occur to us until one workout when we were chatting about how much we hate these intervals and after this month was over we were never parking our butts on those stupid bikes again—that we were *chatting*. While doing the intervals. When we first started with them, we couldn't even reliably produce breath much less words, and here we were completing sentences. Our bodies had acclimated to the intervals. Or we had learned to cheat. Once we realized that we weren't working as hard, we tried just telling ourselves to buckle down and push harder. Whether we'd lost the will to push that hard or our lung capacity had outpaced our leg muscles, I don't know but it lead us to an important conclusion about HIIT: You have to change up the method.

I'm not sure how it was for those forty-five women on bikes now immortalized forever in my mind with glittering halos of sweat and sainthood, but the bikes quickly lost their power to kick our butts. Fortunately HIIT is one of the most adaptable workout programs out there. You can do it with nothing more than running shoes and a stretch of sidewalk, if that's all you have. (Although if you can afford a little more, for the love of humanity, please wear shorts.) Like the fitness Dr. Seuss might say, you can do it with a jump rope, on a rowing machine, in a swimming pool, around a track, or on a treadmill. You can do it in a house! You can do it with a mouse! You can do it (jumping) over a box! You can do it with a fox! I will do them here and there, those intervals—I can do them anywhere!

I was documenting my daily insanity on my blog, and a reader who happened to be a competitive sprinter sent me an evil little workout called a Zoomer. For those of you masochists, this is how a Zoomer looks in theory:

1. While straddling the treadmill, set it to level twelve (5:30 minute miles).
2. Jump on and run like mad for ten seconds.
3. Increase the incline to five. Run for ten seconds.
4. Increase the incline again to ten. Run for ten seconds.
5. Drop down to zero incline and level six (10 minute miles). Run for ten seconds.
6. That's one Zoomer. Repeat.

Charlotte's tip: At least for the first time, have someone else do all the button pushing for you. Just make sure that whomever you pick doesn't secretly hate you.

And here's how a Zoomer looks in practice:

"**ALLISON:** *No.*

ME: *We can totally do this.*

ALLISON: *No.*

Me: *We have to try it.*

Allison: *I cannot run that fast. I'm going to eat it.*

Me: *You will not. We run that fast when we sprint around the track.*

Allison: *No we don't.*

Me: *Well, we did that one time.*

Allison: *Fine. You go first.*

Me: *(feeling the fear of looking down between my feet at an insanely spinning treadmill belt) Do you promise to pick me up if I become a flesh-colored skid mark?*

Allison: *Only after I'm done laughing.*

Me: *Fine.*"

We then proceeded to watch the spinning belts for about ten minutes, occasionally testing it with one shoe, like a swimmer would toe the water. People stared. Finally, I jumped on the treadmill. The first step or two were rocky, but I quickly hit my stride and realized that 5:30 minute miles look a lot faster than they feel. Much heartened, I turned to encourage Allison. Anyone who has ever used a treadmill knows that it is a deadly error to turn your head to the side while running (or drink out of an open-top water bottle or pick up a dropped towel). So just as Allison was giving me one last eye roll and jumping on, I shot off the back of the tready like a human cannonball. Allison, whether out of fear of repeating my feat or just because she routinely underestimates her own strength, soon realized that she can run faster than level twelve. A lot faster. She overran the belt and smacked into the front rail, which threw her backwards. Now there were two skid marks. Our completely unmanned treadmills cried victory. The man jogging next to us giggled. Yes, *giggled.*

Never fear, though: We learned our lessons and jumped right back on that pony, eventually working up to completing three in a row. Although, predictably, that would not be the last time I was publicly humiliated by a treadmill.

Out of the Gym

AN INTERESTING THING HAPPENED during this short-n-fast Experiment. I, the cardio queen, was slowly realizing that not only could I maintain my fitness level, but I could improve it while doing substantially less cardio. For someone who once trained for an entire marathon in a month (more on that in the Double Cardio Experiment in chapter 2) and was used to logging at least thirty miles a week running, this was big news. Like many things in life—money, fame, Jell-O—it turns out that more is not necessarily better.

This concept of less quantity but higher intensity in workouts has been the basis of many of my Experiments (see the chapters on the Primal Blueprint, Functional Fitness, and CrossFit), flying in the face of much of the fitness world's conventional wisdom. After all, what does every woman do when she wants to drop a few pounds? (Besides looking up Master Cleanse on the Internet in a moment of temporary insanity?) She runs. Or walks. Or bikes. Or ellipticizes. She does the Almighty Cardio. And she does it for a long time. But perhaps this is not the best method.

Best Moment

"**Allison:** *Ew! Who spilled their water bottle all over the floor?*

Me: (staring down at the large puddle around my bike) *Nobody. I think that's my sweat.*

Allison: *All of it?*

Me: *Yes. I sweat like a dude.*

Allison: (after a long pause) *You had curry for dinner.*"

The Results

According to my heart rate monitor, I burned an average of 460 calories per twenty-minute workout. I have never before or since got than many calories in that short of a time frame, which speaks both to the fat-burning and vomit-inducing powers of this workout. I dropped 1.5 percent body fat in thirty days. And the strangest result: My resting heart rate (measured during the morbidly named corpse pose in yoga) dropped to 42. From a physiological standpoint, this Experiment was an unmitigated success! And I don't say that often.

There is one major downside, however. This workout sucks. And I mean it. It's hard and it's painful, which makes it difficult to motivate yourself to do it. But if you can keep the big picture in mind, it will be totally worth it. At the very least, try throwing in a few minutes of HIIT a couple of times a week. Because not only did Australia give us anonymous, fat-burning she-women on bikes, but it is also the land of Russell Crowe and Hugh Jackman (just in case you needed some extra motivation)!

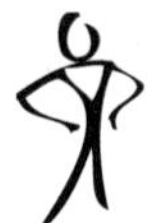

P·E·R·S·O·N·A·L·|·E·S·S·A·Y

My Life As a Cautionary Tale

If I've learned anything from my day job (lie: it's a late-into-the-night job) grading thousands of high school SAT essays—other than that every junior read *The Great Gatsby* this year—it's that life is all about your weaknesses and how you deal with them. Very few seventeen-year-olds are innately good spur-of-the-moment essay writers, and yet the Forces That Be have decreed that if you want to get into a good college, then you'd better be able to crank out something both quasi-meaningful and semi-literate in under thirty minutes. This conundrum forces students to confront one of their weaknesses and deal with it in a high-pressure situation.

Those students who are prepared and/or just talented—about 25 percent by my rough estimation—usually sail through with few problems other than blandness (seriously, I have the most boring job in the world.) It's the rest of the kids who make me alternate between wanting to kill the next texting-at-the-table teen I see in the restaurant and wanting to hug every sad sack in excessive eyeliner and a Hot Topic hoodie. The students unprepared for the exam or perhaps caught up in a clench of testing anxiety usually employ one of several tactics: overconfidence, bluffing, gibberish, or just plain giving up. (Side note: I had a student once who drew me a wonderfully illustrated—yet wordless—cartoon interpretation of the prompt. Sadly, we don't grade for creativity. I still wonder what happened to that kid.) Obviously, the first three irritate me greatly, but it's the last one that breaks my heart. There's usually at least one essay in every batch that is nothing but some eraser marks and tear stains.

Write something! Write anything! I want to scream at them. Even if it's nothing but a tangential recap of last night's *American Idol,* you'll still get some points. But two x-ed out sentences and a damp spot? Nada. You have to at least try.

It makes me think of all the times in my life that I've left nothing but proverbial eraser dribble and tears. I'll be honest: I'm a wuss. I don't have a high pain tolerance or risk tolerance or gore tolerance or any other tolerance. (Back when I was teaching, one of my classes figured out that they could actually get me to run out of the room with my hands over my ears by recounting the plot line to any of the *Saw* movies. My street cred never quite recovered from that one.) I often joke that if I'd been born a serf or a pioneer or a woman in any other age before feminine hygiene products were invented, I probably would have died before passing on my genes, thus ending the Charlotte lineage of crazy before it could even get going.

There is an upside to my wussitude, however. Having so many weaknesses makes me confront them on a regular basis. And this—while painful and often embarrassing—generally makes for a lot of good learning opportunities. Our society tends to focus on individual strengths—encouraging people to hone their skills, focus on their assets, and trumpet their achievements. But here's the thing: The real growth comes not from doing what you already do well, but from trying what you suck at enough times that you get better. There is little interest for me in reading about people who were born good at what they do (um, hi, Lance Armstrong). I'd much rather hear about those who struggle and fight and earn every inch of what they've got. And if I'm being really honest, those are the things I like best about myself.

I take for granted my speed-reading ability because, frankly, I've always been good at that. I've never had to struggle to learn to read. But on the other hand, for years I was painfully, gut-wrenchingly, awkward-as-Daria-on-MTV shy. It's taken me a lot of work and effort (and, yes, reading) to overcome what I had once seen as an unchangeable personality trait, an accomplishment that holds far more value for me. Another weakness that I'm currently working on overcoming is my obsession with and hatred of my body, in particular my weight. It's so omnipresent in my mind that everyone around me is sick of hearing about it. I get tired of writing it. And thinking it and crying over it and wasting time on it. I'm not over it yet. But I'm not going to quit confronting it until I've conquered it. (Jelly bean weakness duly noted. It's on the list too. Somewhere. Bottom-ish.)

This is the problem I have with most fitness stories. It's all about the "Before" (cue frowny face and big lumpy T-shirt) and the "After!" (bring on the fake tan, three-quarter turn and bikini in heels!). So very little is said about the struggle in the middle. It's not that I don't ever want to hear about what people do right—we all need more positivity—but is it wrong to want to hear the messy middle too?

Thanks to advancements in medicine and eugenics laws, a lot of us weak folk are surviving. But life is about so much more than just surviving it. To thrive you have to learn from your weaknesses, whether they be physical, mental, or spiritual. All of which means that at least my life will never be boring.

One of the best things about working out at my particular YMCA is the big "special" bus that rolls up every morning and unloads a group of handicapped people. Some of them sell homemade cards in the lobby, others congregate around the free coffee, but some of them make it onto the fitness floor. This used to frighten me: They make loud noises, monopolize all the exercise balls, and one of them walks around the track swinging his arms as if caught in an invisible gnat cloud at all times. But as I got to know them, and they started to share their accomplishments with me, I came to love them—even the girl who brings all her beanie babies to yoga and lines them up facing her mat. (You try doing down dog with an audience of fifty-one little plastic eyes!)

They have taught me: There is value in fallibility.

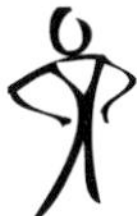

chapter eleven

November
Going Vegan

I HAVE A CONFESSION TO MAKE: I'm partial to Victoria Posh Spice-Beckham. (Is that right? It just feels right to hyphenate that.) I blame it on the fact that the Spice Girls were popular during my crucial formative years. To this day I still have the Latin remix of "Spice Up Your Life" on my iPod. She's so cute and twee! Nobody rocks a pixie cut like that girl. Plus, she has three boys, just like I do. And my husband even loves to play soccer. We'd have a lot to talk about over dinner, is what I'm saying.

So when she showed up—in photos, of course, not on my front doorstep—toting a copy of *Skinny Bitch* by Rory Freedman and Kim Barnouin, I got swept up in the nationwide frenzy. Ignoring the obvious question of why the skinniest woman on earth was trying to get thinner, I decided to go Vegan too for three months. (Note to scientists: if Posh gets any tinier, then she will most likely implode, and you will finally get to study a black hole up close. Score one for science!) Strangers thought I was a poseur, my friends thought I was nuts, and my family thought I had relapsed into my eating disorder. And they were all kind of right.

The Theory

IF YOU ARE UNFAMILIAR WITH THE BOOK, it purports to give The Secret to being thin, fabulous, and envied by all. It's actually an introduction to veganism. With a lot of cursing. Which, if you know anything about vegans, should not surprise you. The book comes complete with enough animal cruelty horror stories to make PETA proud. This might have put some people off the diet right away, but as I'd been a vegetarian on and off for years, it sounded kinda fun. Some people claim they felt betrayed by the authors' hidden agenda. I say if hidden agendas in the diet industry surprise you, then you should probably stay away from haunted houses. And fun houses. And probably friends' houses as well. Just in case they inadvertently surprise you.

The rules to the vegan game are simple: no animal products. Obviously this means no meat, dairy, eggs, or fish. However, you will quickly learn that there are many other things that fall under the animal umbrella. Jell-O, for instance, is made from cow hooves (I know, I'm sorry, but someone had to tell you). Leather shoes, belts, and dominatrix collars are also frowned upon. Tongue piercings, though, are iffy—while they are metal and therefore not made of animal butts, I don't know that anyone in good conscience could call them "cruelty free." I'm still waiting for Alicia Silverstone to get back to me on that one. Even sugar, as it is traditionally processed using bone char from dead animals (or humans—I don't know how picky they are), can be problematic. And don't even get me started on the Great Vegan Honey Debate, although it does make for entertaining cocktail party conversation. Here, I'll get you started: Are bees animals? Does their butt juice constitute an animal product? Do bees die in the process of making honey or are the dead bees just old or infirm? Discuss.

Anyhow, I decided to keep my knee-high sexy boots—every girl needs a pair of sexy boots—and just focus on the food aspect. Now, those of you that are thinkers have already realized that a diet of French fries (fried in vegetable oil) and diet Coke is vegan. While you would be correct, the Skinny Bitches put the kibosh on that right away by adding that you need to cut out alcohol, caffeine, sugar, and junk food.

The Diet

My first shopping trip as a vegan can best be described as a religious experience. I felt clean and pure as I walked righteously past the meat counter, the dairy case, and all those aisles and aisles of boxed stuff. When I accidentally knocked a low-lying bag of Cheetos off a shelf, I couldn't bear to pick it up with my sanctified fingers. I was holy.

I was also starving. I came home with a few grocery bags of produce, some soy milk, one loaf of frozen Ezekiel bread—so few people buy it in Minnesota that the only place I could find it was frozen in the Expensive Foods Store—and a vegan pizza that did not look at all appetizing. Oh, and a few boxes of veggie burgers.

Over the first few weeks, the authors' claims of rapid weight loss were born out as I watched the scale go down. But that was mostly because I just didn't know what to eat. I'd stand in front of the refrigerator with a bewildered look on my face until I'd either eat another veggie burger or wander away in frustration. As I slowly got the hang of what I could and couldn't eat, however, it got easier to plan complete meals and my weight stabilized. I had a decent repertoire of meals I could cook and that tasted pretty good. Well, at home anyhow.

Eating out was an entirely different story. Being vegan in our society is a very difficult thing to do. Unless you live in California or Manhattan, which I do not. Friends would invite us over for dinner, and I then either had to explain all my food restrictions and hope they could come up with something tasty we could all eat, or I had to eat beforehand and feign stomach cramps when I got to their house. Being a non-evangelizing vegan, I generally chose the latter route, which led to many uncomfortable conversations ending in "Just eat something already!" Restaurants were even worse. Ordering was a twenty-minute process during which the poor waiter got bombarded with more questions than Britney Spears after she shaved her head (may her weave rest in peace). I remember going out for Mexican with some very good friends and ending up with a tiny cup of plain black beans while everyone else devoured pollo enchiladas and sopa con queso. My holiness was devolving into bitterness.

The net result was that I just stopped going out to functions that involved food. Normally a very social person, this self-imposed isolation started to take a toll. In the book, the authors talk about hosting large vegan parties or going out to eat with all their vegan friends. It was then I realized that they suffer from the California delusion.

The Coastal Food Divide

California exports health and fitness advice like China exports lead-covered baby toys. And, most of the time, said advice can be generalized to the public at large. However, I sometimes think that all the personal trainers and health gurus forget that many of us don't live in the land of eternal sunshine (aka the place where food actually grows on trees).

It's not just that the tanned and toned ignore our inability to run outside in a minus thirty-five-degree windstorm or the fact that the local grocery store thinks purslane is a new line of designer handbags made just for Target. It's that they overlook the differences in the entire food culture.

I moved to the Midwest from Seattle—a place where you can get organic produce at the farmer's market year-round and salmon right off the boat. (Oh, and that nonsense about it raining all the time? Lies to keep all the rest of you from moving there. New York gets more rain than Seattle.) I never knew how good I had it until

I moved here and discovered tiny, shriveled apples on "sale" for $2.49 a pound.

Don't get me wrong, I absolutely love it here. People on the street actually meet your eyes and say hi. And not just tinfoil-hatted crazies! Normal people will talk to you in the checkout lane. Teenagers hold doors open for grandmas. There's a playground on every corner. And the local Honeycrisp apples, when they are in season, are the closest thing to Apple Heaven I've ever come (even if they do still sell for $2.49 a pound). But if I were to follow the current food craze to "eat local," it'd be snow cones and sausage six months out of the year.

In addition to the physical limitations, there is also a prevailing food culture here. I hesitate to bring it up lest I conjure perverse images of *Fargo* or *America's Next Top Model* and thus blaspheme against my new and much-loved home, but it is the simple truth. The PTA here opens the year with a beer-n-brat tent. Almost every birthday party my children are invited to is in a fast food establishment. All fish comes fried. Hotdish (read: casserole based around Campbell's Cream-o-whatever) is the regional delicacy and shows up at every function. The schools hand out Pizza Hut certificates for reading, McDonald's Happy Meals for math, and Culver's Custard (ice cream) for playing sports. And we have one of the highest rates of drunk driving in the country.

As much as we like to believe in a TV-homogenized America, there simply is a difference between the way people on the coasts and people in the middle think about food. Disclaimer: The one place I've never lived is in the South, so I can't speak to their food culture, but if Paula Deen is any indication, it is about as far from the Cali-sushi-veg aesthetic as you can get and still stay in our borders.

Why is it that we can accept that the French and the Italians and the Swedes each have their own way of eating and yet fail to see and appreciate the differences in our own country? I expect that some of you will answer (or at least think), "Well, it's because the Europeans are trim and healthy, whereas somebody better put you Americans out to pasture before milking time."

And yet, as of 2008, Minneapolis is the second healthiest city in the nation for the fourth year in a row! That's right, somehow it all balances out—the vicious weather, the McDonald's birthdays, the freaking hotdish. We exercise indoors. We take vitamin D tablets. We eat a lot of frozen fruits and veggies. (Bonus: You don't even need an extra freezer here! Just throw it out your back door.) We make it work, but it ain't the California way.

The Workout

THE FITNESS PORTION OF THE BOOK WAS VERY SHORT. Basically the authors say to do it—although they don't really tell you what kind or how long or not to wear gray cotton shorts because they will show your crotch sweat (you're welcome!)—but not to get too crazy about it. Then they both sort of 'fess up that they're not really into exercising and getting your diet straight is really the most important part. And they may be right about that. Most health and fitness professionals say that 70–80 percent of health and weight maintenance is about nutrition, with only 20–30 percent being about fitness.

The problem is that doesn't work so well for me. I enjoy working out. I *love* it. In fact, sometimes I love it so much that it has to tell me we need to take a break and see other people and for the love of little green apples stop calling all the time or the police will get involved. The Skinny Bitches—both being former fashion models complete with model DNA—may not need to exercise, but I sure do. The SB girls also recommend that you eat a very light breakfast, consisting solely of fruit. This did not sound like a good idea for me, as I do most of my workouts in the morning, but being the good lab rat that I am, I had fruit for breakfast for two weeks.

In the Gym

THE FIRST DAY I WAS SO DIZZY I had to leave my kickboxing class and sit down. An old man asked me if I was pregnant. Yeah, not what I was going for. The next day I almost fell off my Spin bike, which would have been doubly painful as my shoes were stuck in those little cage things on the pedals. After that, I adapted by eating a huge meal right before bed just so I could have enough energy to work out the next morning, from which I learned that I don't sleep well when I eat a huge meal right before bed. As soon as the two weeks were up, I was back to my daily a.m. food fests.

Results

By the end of my three-month Experiment, I was pleasantly surprised to discover that except for the loss of eggs and cheese, I did rather enjoy eating vegan. I liked that I wasn't eating animals and that I was helping save the planet and that now I had an official reason to never ever eat hot dogs again. Eliminating sugar was difficult, but I did like how I felt, although I doubted my ability to stay away from the White Satan forever. (Indeed, two years post-Experiment, I'm fully back on the jelly beans.)

As far as my weight was concerned, after the initial loss due to my confusion about what to eat, there was no more. Here's the thing about veganism: You can cheat on it. Just like Atkins followers learn how to get around the no-carb rule by eating tons of bad-for-you chocolate "protein" bars, vegans can cheat too. A vegan pizza still has a white-bread crust and is loaded with fat. A vegan cookie is still packed with sugar even if it's hidden under the guise of "brown rice syrup." Once you get used to being vegan, I think you still have all the struggles of people on a more conventional diet except that you are ten times as annoying to waiters.

The other result of my vegan Experiment was the reemergence of my past eating disorder, but this time in a new form. I got so caught up in eating just the "right" foods, that I ended up orthorexic (a made-up name for a new eating disorder where people are obsessed with eating healthy—ironically, to the detriment of their own health) and landed on ABC's *20/20* as their freak show of the week (see chapter 4).

While I can't blame the Skinny Bitches or veganism in general for this as my disordered eating tendencies were pre-existing, I do think that disordered eaters are more attracted to very

Worst Moment

THE SETTING: Thanksgiving Day at my long-suffering parents' house.

MOM: *Since I know you are a vegetarian or whatever, I made sure to make you some special food! There are mashed potatoes, they don't have meat . . .*

ME: *Um, I can't eat butter or milk.*

MOM: *Oh, okay! Well I got you a Tofurkey! It's so funny—it even looks like meat!*

ME: *I can't eat Tofurkey either.*

MOM: *Why not?*

ME: *Processed soy gives me horrible gas.*

MOM: *That explains you as an infant then. Soy formula! No wonder you were such a difficult baby. Anyhow, here's some Jell-O!*

ME: *Cow hooves, Mom.*

MOM: *What?*

ME: *Jell-O isn't vegan. Gelatin is made from collagen rendered from boiling bones, hooves, and skins of animals.*

MOM: *Well, that's pleasant.*

[Uncomfortable silence]

DAD: *So you're going to eat salad then?*

ME: *After I brush the cheese off of it.*

To their immense credit, no one smacked me that day. It wasn't long afterward that I realized that I had a problem if I couldn't even eat dinner with my family.

restrictive diets than "normal" people. Of all the vegans that I have met over the years, I'd guess at least half have some kind of diagnosable eating disorder.

In the end, after much therapy and fights over food with my family, I downgraded to "just" a non-militant vegetarian who sometimes eats fish.

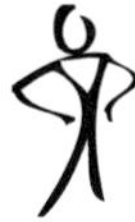

P·E·R·S·O·N·A·L·|·E·S·S·A·Y

Field Notes from an Orthorexic

In talking about orthorexia, I hear the same comments over and over again. The thing that seems to confuse people most about the unofficial eating disorder is how one can be so concerned with eating healthy and end up so unhealthy. So, in the interest of public service, here's my step-by-step guide on how to be as messed up as I was:

Step One—Find Research that Sounds Authoritative

For me it started with a sincere desire to "get healthy." Sadly, I had no idea what that meant. I'd grown up, like many of my peers, on white-bread sandwiches with processed cheese followed by a Little Debbie chaser. Adding peach slices in heavy syrup made it healthy, not to mention rounding out the "orange" theme on my plate. In home ec class (yeah, they actually had one in my high school, and I actually took it), we learned essential skills, like how to fold cloth napkins into a bird and how to sew the legs of your drawstring pants together but zilch about nutrition. College was the height of my eating disorder, so my menus were entertaining little tidbits like *one fun-size package of Chewy Gobstoppers. Per day.* Occasionally I'd mix it up with Lipton Rice & Sauce. I remember one time my roommate brought home a twenty-pound box of orchard fresh apples. We ate that entire box in two days, so starved for produce we were. Obviously, I needed help.

Thankfully, in this day and age, nutritive help abounds. I read every book, Web site, and magazine article I could get my hands on. For instance, take this little gem about milk: Lose Four Times The Fat and Build Twice the Muscle Drinking Milk! (I made that title up, but it encapsulates a whole slew of research that came out around this time.)

Step Two—Implement Advice

The study sounds believable. But then, they almost always do—at least to me. My love of research is probably one of my worst orthorexic weaknesses. Even the best study is not infallible and I know it but, those researchers, they always sound so sure of themselves! And they're smart! And I'm losing IQ points by the child! So I do what they say. In this case, drink a cup of milk post workout.

Step Three—Find Contradictory Research

If there is anything researchers love more than research (and forwarding arcane insider jokes to each other over their university intranets), it is contradicting other researchers' research. Nothing grabs headlines like refuting a popular study. In fact, I hear Britney was almost bumped from her number one Google spot by those Women's Health Initiative people. Okay, not true but it should be. For example, this study: Milk Studies Misleading—Milk Does Not Aid in Weight Loss. This one is particularly good because it manages to refute *all* milk studies at the same time. Genius!

Step Four—Get Confused

Since I trust other people's knowledge, particularly science-y types, more than my own, I am left in a quandary. Milk is da bomb! Milk sucks! Milk chocolate often has no actual milk in it! So what am I to do?

Step Five—Try Logic

By far the worst step. Some people try and cheat past this step by just blindly following a particular diet like South Beach or Atkins or Mariah Carey's purple bender. Sheep! At this point, I would try and figure out the flaws of each study. Sample sizes? Research institution? Funding source? Duration of test? Longitudinal? Case study? Self report? Were twins involved? Animals? Ouija boards?

Okay, so maybe all milk isn't bad. If I go up a dollar on the price scale, there's the no-hormone milk. But it's not organic. Another dollar gets me organic but not from grass-fed cows. Another dollar gets me grass (oh, the joke I could make here about the street value of cow juice compared to marijuana these days but I'm too busy being neurotic—excuse me while I continue getting worked up). And then there's the whole issue of are the cows just finished on grass or actually grass fed their entire doomed lives? And is the grass organic? Another dollar up—now about twelve dollars a half gallon—gets you organic, antibiotic-free, hormone-free, free-range, unpasteurized, unhomogenized, and totally grassed-up cows. But . . . I can't afford that!

Besides, cows are the single biggest contributor of methane—a greenhouse gas four times worse than CO_2. And cows pollute ground water. And eat up valuable land that could be used to grow food for starving Africans. And cows are named cute things like Bessie and Daisy. Not to mention everyone says that dairy makes you bloat.

Step Six—Make Arbitrary Rule

Once you're this far down the crazy path, you either let your brain explode or you have to decide something. Fine. There's just too much uncertainty. Milk is out.

Step Seven—Repeat

Now repeat steps one through six for eggs, meat, soy, nuts, seeds, fruits, tubers, leafy vegetables, cheese, bread, sugar, artificial sweeteners, boxed cereals, canned produce, frozen produce, juice, microwave meals, grains, caffeine . . . ad nauseum.

Which is exactly how I got to the point where all I ate were green veggies, some fruits, and nuts. Congratulations—you're a squirrel! Welcome to the nut house.

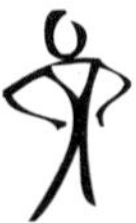

chapter twelve

December
Karate

THERE ARE SOME EXPERIMENTS that end up being about so much more than the gym. I can honestly say that this Experiment changed my life. As a naïve college student, I was mentally and sexually abused by my boyfriend at the time. For four years after our breakup, I ignored the darkness that clawed inside me, but it all broke loose when he was arrested for sexually assaulting two other girls. As the victim count rose, my mental state plummeted. After a protracted court case in which I was a key witness, he was finally sent to prison. In the TV version I would have emerged vindicated, empowered, and whole again as Mariska Hargitay hugged me and told me I did a great thing.

Instead, I was deeply broken. Nothing about it, not even the final sentencing, had felt good or right. If anything, I felt even more vulnerable than before. I had not expected a Great Fitness Experiment to be the key to finally start healing that trauma.

But it did. Sometimes life surprises you.

"I want to kill people," I informed Sensei Don Seiler at our first meeting in his tiny basement dojo. It is to his credit that he hardly blinked. Perhaps it comes with the territory of being a third-degree black belt or maybe Gym Buddy Megan—his wife—warned him about me first, but either way he took it all in stride. "With all due respect," I continued, "I realize that Karate is a martial art, but I'm less interested in the art and more in the martial." Because if you start a sentence with "with all due respect" that means the other person can't get offended, right? I've seen *The Karate Kid*; there would be no wax on/wax off nonsense for this girl.

"Fine," he nodded. "Ever heard of Ikken Hissatsu? It means one punch, one kill." Mr. Miyagi he was not.

I got giddy. I'll admit it. Ever since I started The Great Fitness Experiment, various readers have been encouraging me to do a Martial Arts Experiment of some sort. And given its reputation for being a hard-core, full-body workout, I was eager to give it a try. Plus, and I swear I'm not a total psychopath, I really like to hit people, and I never get to do it—something about it not being a socially acceptable habit or whatever. Sensei Don let me down quickly though. Apparently, to reliably kill people (as opposed to an accident in a bar fight, which is called a one-punch homicide and will land you in jail, where, if you are really lucky, you can write a rap song about it and make a million bucks, but barring that, you will live out the rest of your days being miserable and lonely, so don't do it), you have to be, well, good at karate. And being good at karate means learning all the basic forms.

The Theory

As Sensei Don informed me, they call it a martial "art" for a reason: It's not just about fighting; it's about training the mind, body, and character to work together for self protection. Ideally, it's mostly about strengthening the mind, and character and the body will follow suit. In practice, it means that you start with the most rudimentary techniques—called standing basics—and perform them hundreds of times until they become ingrained. In addition, you perform routines of these basics—called kata—hundreds of times to demonstrate your mastery. And in case you get bored easily, you also get to yell a lot. When I expressed my worry about yelling in the gym and looking crazy, Gym Buddy Megan cracked up something fierce. That girl.

There was more hilarity to be had once I got to the gym the following Monday to introduce the Matsubayashi Ryu Karate-Do Experiment.

"Okay, everyone get warmed up because today we start our new Karate Experiment." Holding up two small pieces of wood, I continued in my most serious voice, "We will begin by breaking these boards."

You should have seen the Gym Buddies' faces! Until Gym Buddy Megan busted up laughing. Again. But I had Gym Buddy Allison good and scared for about half a second.

Actually, the blocks of wood were there for a painful purpose. Sensei Don gave them to me to toughen up my knuckles. You know, so it won't hurt so much when I punch stuff. He instructed me to do two sets of thirty push-ups a day. On the wood boards. *On my knuckles.*

Allison was not down with this. "

"**ALLISON:** *But it hurts!"*

ME: *"It's supposed to hurt,"* I answered. I did one knuckle push-up.

ALLISON: *"It hurts a lot!"*

ME: *"I know!"* Two knuckle push-ups.

ALLISON: *"I have girly hands!"*

ME: *"Me too."* Three knuckle push-ups.

ALLISON: *"It's easier if you do it this way."* She turned her hands to the side.

ME: *"Ow, ow, ow, ow... okay."*"

It took me three measly knuckle push-ups before I gave up and finished out the set the normal way. We threatened Megan with Ikken Hissatsu if she told on us. She laughed hysterically. Well, at least she was getting a good ab workout.

The Workout

SENSEI DON DEVISED A WORKOUT broken up into three major parts for us: conditioning, standing basics, and kata. He instructed us to spend an hour a day on these things and then do whatever we wish with the rest of our time (helllooo cardio!).

Conditioning

The main parts to focus on for karate are your core, legs, forearms, and back. He said that to be effective at karate we need to learn to rely less on our chest and biceps and more on using gravity and our body weight to help us punch and kick. So we were to do one hundred reps of crunches, leg raises (the ab kind, not the Jane Fonda kind), one minute of supermans (where you lie on your stomach and pretend you're flying except that your stunt cable broke, and you don't know it yet), and squats.

Standing Basics

The easiest way to learn these is to have a qualified sensei teach them to you. However, if you can't find one or are as cheap as I am, you can always get Sensei Don's book *Karate-Do: Traditional Training for All Styles styles* by Kevin Seiler and Donald Seiler (www.kodokan-seiler.com). I tell you what, the book is worth it just for the photos—that man knows how to look fierce in a picture. Miss Tyra ain't got nothing on Sensei Don.

There are about twenty standing basics of which beginners only practice the first ten or so. But repeating each of those one hundred times took the better part of an hour, and I was pretty tight in my shoulders and sweaty by the time we were done.

Kata

The best way to describe the kata is that it is like a dance. Except a really tough guy dance. With yelling. Take a few standing basics, mix them up with some random turning and stepping, add a few "kee-ahs!" and there you have it. If you are interested in seeing them done right, there are plenty of videos on the Internet with guys in sharp, white gis (prounced gee, with a hard g). If you want a good giggle, the Gym Buddies and I are YouTube kata stars.

Out of the Gym

MY FIRST INDICATION THAT THIS WOULD NOT BE MY AVERAGE Experiment came the night after my first Karate lesson. I don't know if it was the imposing, all-seeing eye of Bob—the grimacing torso on a stick that Karate students use to practice their kicks, punches, and cheap groin shots—or just the general trauma brought on by being a victim of violence trying to learn to be violent herself, but I had nightmares of my sexual assault all night.

One phrase from Sensei Don in particular had lodged itself in my mind. It was in response to a question I asked if one could train killer instinct or if he—and karate philosophy—believe it is inborn. He replied, "About 98 percent of people are sheep. You put them in a situation where it's life or death, such as the random knife attack on the bus in Canada (where a crazy man stabbed, killed, and beheaded a fellow passenger while the rest of the people on the bus just watched), and most people will run away or hide. The remaining 2 percent—the wolves—have the instinct to fight."

"So how does one know if they have the instinct to fight or not?" I had asked.

"You don't. Until it's tested."

I was tested once.

The night I was sexually assaulted, I was asleep. So he had the element of surprise on his side, not to mention an extra sixty pounds and nine inches. But I really think that it was the sleep that got me. The prosecutor would later make an assertion that I had been drugged, but whether it was a chemically induced stupor or just shock, I woke up slowly. Too slowly. In my groggy state, it took me even longer to realize what was going on.

Despite the fact that he had a weapon—if you can call a razor blade a weapon—it didn't feel particularly violent. Although later when I was cleaning up, I would marvel at my torn clothing and the blood. But it wasn't my blood; it was his. You see, the blade was meant to get me to comply but not by killing me but rather by threatening to kill himself. Looking back I'm sure he didn't mean it, that it was just one of many ways he manipulated me that night. But at the time, I was sure he did mean it, and I had already come to the conclusion that one of us was going to die at his hand.

At the time, it felt like it took forever, but in reality I think it was over fairly quickly. I remember that I tried screaming but gave that up when I realized that no one could hear me and it only antagonized him. So I cried instead. Just a quiet steady river that ran into my hair and down my neck. The great gulping sobs, along with the uncontrollable shaking, wouldn't come until hours later when I was safe. And alone. When the physical-ness of it was over, the real drama began. He raved and whispered, cursed me and caressed me, threatened and pleaded. I watched from inside myself. And then I drove him home.

Not once did I fight him.

Aside from resisting as he removed my clothing, I was consumed by a sort of helpless passivity. Inevitability. Instinct, if you will. Others have since told me that I did what my mind thought was safest at the time and that I shouldn't judge myself for (not) doing what I did. But it haunts me, that thing I didn't do. I didn't even try to fight him. He would not have killed me.

When I finally discovered kickboxing years later, it seemed the perfect antidote to the vulnerability that plagued me. I have convinced myself that were I to ever find myself in a similar situation, this time I would fight back. I would not again willingly become a victim.

But what if that is not true? What if I lacked that instinct of self-preservation? Not only had I proven myself a sheep once, but thanks to the horrors of the post-traumatic stress disorder (PTSD) that consumed me during the court case, I have demonstrated over and over again that what I do is duck and cringe. And scream.

Without even stepping foot in a gym or a dojo, I was discovering how difficult it was going to be for me to do this Karate Experiment without facing the specter that introduced me to the desire to punch and kick in the first place. I do not take well to being handled by other people. I react strongly to innocent touch and overreact to aggressive touch. I tried once, years ago, to take a self-defense class, but I made the mistake of doing a mixed-gender class, and I ended it early in tears, feeling molested.

The questions that haunted me that first night: Is it possible to change from a sheep to a fox? Are these patterns ingrained or can they be retrained? Could I be a fighter if I had the will but lacked the instinct?

In The Gym

THE NEXT DAY AT THE YMCA, Gym Buddy Vernie, a competitive Muay Thai kickboxer who is built like a brick wall, sensed that something in me had changed. Without me even having to say a word, he brought out his kickboxing gloves and showed me how to wrap my hands in them. They felt heavy but more secure than my untrained bare hands—a liability in karate and not just in regards to knuckle pushups. He told me to punch him in the arm. I pulled a girl. I know. It's so lame I can barely write about it. At first I giggled and only threw weak badly aimed jabs. But he kept encouraging me—egging me on really—to hit him harder and harder until I was throwing a punch with all the aggression I could muster. "Good," he said once I was all punched out, "now you just need to learn how to put your body weight behind the throw. Hips, shoulder, then fist."

It felt really good and not just because he told Allison that she punched like a wuss (she was too polite). Pregnant Gym Buddy

Megan, on the other hand, was a powerhouse. Call it instinct or those Mama Bear hormones, but I would not want to come down on the wrong side of that girl in a dark alley.

My next moment of Karate-induced Zen didn't come until several weeks later. Anyone who has worked out in a gym setting knows that there is such a thing as gym politics. You remember those people from middle school—you know, the ones who dropped a sloppy joe in your super-cool Esprit bag or hawked a loogie in your super-cool '80's bangs? (What? Was that just me?) Well it turns out that many of them grew up to work in the fitness profession. Perhaps it is their undying love of their cheerleader shorts and the desire to always fit in them or just a fetish for watching other people in pain, but I'm convinced a disproportionate number of mean kids grow up to be personal trainers. Although, in a way, middle school was easier, because then I wasn't burdened with the knowledge that they are actual human beings. It turns out they have handicapped kids and abusive husbands and car problems and the insatiable wedgie that became unavoidable when thongs became *the* fitness underwear du jour. Basically they're still jerks. It's just harder to hate them for it.

Anyhow, I was having a highly irritating, energy-sucking, completely eighth grade spat with one queen bee that was interfering with my daily sweat fests by turning them into daily whine-to-the-Gym-Buddies-while-we-run-endless-laps fests. True to middle-school form, it even reduced me to tears one night after a particularly caustic comment.

And then, like Jiminy Cricket but with much hairier arms, Sensei Don appeared in my mind. At our last lesson he had taught

Gym Buddy Allison and me a game called "Sticky Hands." It involves standing with your wrists "glued" together, palms up. Then you move your arms in synch with your partner. If they throw a punch, you just follow them, gently moving their arm away. The goal is to get the other person to move their feet first. Sensei Don, needing to get some humor out of this since we weren't paying him, let us do this for several rounds—which ended up looking like we were playing imaginary Twister whilst standing up and giggling an unseemly amount—before telling us the trick. It goes back to that whole gravity-is-a-law-of-nature thing people keep telling me about: when someone punches at you, you gently pull them toward you thereby using their momentum to unbalance them. Same thing if they pull you—you gently push toward them until they take a step.

We didn't have much luck doing it in practice, mostly because Allison and I are way too polite—"You go first!" "No, you go first!" "Okay, I'm going to punch now, are you ready?" But the thought rang particularly relevant for my fight with the Gym Class President. Because what was our struggle if not a push-pull playground tug-of-war? And so it became. Over the next few weeks, when she pushed, I pulled her closer to me. When she pulled me, I leaned in. At first I thought that giving up the control of the argument to her would make me lose, but as I watched her initial surprise and then acceptance of my kindness, it was apparent I was on to something. The bratty eighth grader in me immediately thought of how I could manipulate my newfound power to bend her to my will, but then I realized that would ruin my whole new grown-up mojo. I let go completely.

And the fight de-escalated to the point of unremarkability. Not only was I relieved to be left in peace, but the Gym Buddies were thrilled that I had regained my ability to converse about other more important topics, such as why thongs are *the* fitness underwear du jour.

The Results

As the Karate Experiment wore on, I discovered that I actually enjoy doing the kata—that there is beauty in the details. At the beginning this was the part I wanted most to skip over in my Karate training. And yet because Sensei Don told us it was important to learn, the Gym Buddies and I did our best to squelch our silliness and practiced it faithfully several times a day. (Although we may have broken out into Rockette kicks on a few occasions. It couldn't be helped.)

Then one day I realized I liked it. There was a sense of mastery in remembering the order and I felt amazingly accomplished the first time we all got it right. (There was screaming and a few cheerleader jumps. No chest bumping though—Gym Buddy Megan was pregnant, remember?) But the moment when I truly realized its worth was when we performed it for Sensei Don. He stepped in and showed us what we had really learned: a sequence of moves that was not arbitrary, like I had thought, but was designed to block and attack a certain offense. And when I did it right, it worked! In all the self-defense classes I've taken, I've never actually ended up with a move that really worked. And now I had three! I was positively giddy. I went home and tried them on my husband. They worked on him too! That is until he decided to just throw me over his shoulder and tickle me until I threatened to pee on him. Incidentally, that last technique, dubbed the Turtle, isn't covered in self-defense books, but I've had good results with it.

The last thing that I learned was that unrestrained emotion hurts. Never before have I ever felt so very fragile during an Experiment. And I think it made me stronger. Karate is good therapy.

The first time I felt this strength was during one of the first lessons when Sensei Don asked if he could touch my throat. He had no way of knowing that that is my panic spot. Even now just thinking about it makes my heart pound and the bile rise in my throat. I don't let anyone touch my neck, not even my children. My response was to throw Gym Buddy Megan under the bus. "Can you do it on her?" Sensei Don replied that he would, but he wanted me to feel where the pressure points on the neck were. And so I said yes. And you know what? I was okay. Not great—I did tear up a bit, but I don't think anyone noticed—but I was okay. And now I know that about myself.

The second time was much more dramatic. After all those weeks of drills, Sensei Don finally deemed us ready to punch something. So he got out his pads and showed us a drill where we did two punches and a block as hard as we could for two minutes straight. Now, I have *done* interval training. And I will tell you that this was some of the highest intensity interval training that I have ever done. It had something that sprinting does not though: I got to hit stuff. Within just a few punches, I discovered the satisfying thrill of smashing my hand into something—hard. It felt really good. In fact, it felt so good that I didn't realize until after the first interval was over that my left hand had two split knuckles, and I was about to leave blood spatter in the dojo. I quickly taped it up though because I didn't want to miss my next interval, and Sensei Don was not stopping the clock for me.

For some reason that I still can't fully explain, all that punching did something to me. Like my knuckles, something inside me split open, and while it hurt, it felt good to get it out. I cried when I got home, and it wasn't because of the pain in my hands (although, seriously, that hurt! I do not recommend splitting your knuckles). Afterwards, I felt lighter than I had in a really long time. It was a high that didn't leave me for days. I even dreamt about installing my own makiwara (a leather punching/kicking post) in my basement so I could do it again.

I learned that those tides of emotions that overwhelm me at times can be controlled without repressing them. That I can experience them without being consumed by them.

Conclusion

So how was Karate as a workout? That was the original point of this Experiment, right? It was fairly rigorous. Like many workouts, it is as hard as you make it. Sensei Don kept things tough for us by having us do daily conditioning exercises like push-ups (including on our knuckles), sit-ups, and squats. At his dojo he came up with some circuit training that involved functional weight

Best Moment

Despite having a high school boyfriend who used to punch bricks for fun (don't worry, we broke up), I had never had the pleasure of pounding something until I was a bloody pulp before. Punching pads held by Sensei Don was such a rush that I didn't even realize my knuckles were bleeding until it was all over, and I noticed the blood on the backs of my hands. The adrenaline was so crazy that I didn't even feel the pain! Some will say that is how childbirth is, but I beg to differ—having birthed five of the little nippers myself, I can tell you categorically that nothing dampens the pain of natural childbirth. Also? You totally don't forget. Anyhow, I was so excited after taping up my knuckles that I had to take a picture of my bruised and battered hands and text them to everyone I knew. Unfortunately, my movie moment was over the next day when I woke up with hands so stiff and sore I could barely hold a pencil. And those scabs took weeks to heal. I'd do it again in a heartbeat.

exercises specific to the Karate movements that we were training. And, of course, the repeated punches and kicks could definitely bring on a good sweat. We added some free weights and cardio of our own as well as daily standing basics and kata drills. Despite never targeting specific muscle groups with our Karate training, I found that my shoulders and upper arms got some additional muscle definition.

Karate was definitely one of my favorite Experiments. Generally, as the Gym Buddies and I get to the end of the month, it gets harder to motivate ourselves to do the workout. We're ready to be done and move on to the next thing. This time, however, I wished I had more time to continue it. One month was simply not enough to learn everything that I want to know about Karate. This will be one activity that I will keep up with even though the thirty days are up. Gotta get my punching fix in somehow!

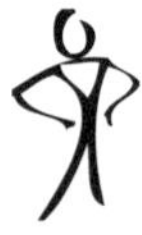

P·E·R·S·O·N·A·L | ·E·S·S·A·Y

$5.24

I am the only person I know who regularly gets money in the mail and hates it. The envelope gives it away. If it was from Publishers Clearing House and was the size of an ice cream truck, I might feel differently, but the letter today is from the State Department of Corrections, Offender Obligation Unit. I don't want to open it. The girl who takes karate lessons and punches until her knuckles bleed wants to just rip it into a thousand tiny pieces and throw them into the spring wind to catch in somebody's lawn and eventually be made into a nest. But the practical part of me needs to know. I tell myself that I need to open it because there may be important information in there, like when his parole is up and if he'll get his name off the sex-offender registry and if he's moved to my state or reoffended or . . . What I really want to know is how much I'm worth.

Today I'm worth $5.24.

Back when the verdict was rendered and the plea was bargained and the sentence was imposed, nothing was said to me of money. That came later when my victim's advocate asked me for my receipts. "Receipts for what?" I asked. The State had paid for my plane ticket to testify, and I'd stayed with my brother and his wife. I hadn't even incurred any food costs as I was too white-knuckled black-curtained panicked to eat. "Oh, he is going to pay you some money, dear," she answered cheerfully. "Certainly you have expenses he has caused." Can you put a price on mental anguish?

He offered to pay me, once.

"You're making too big a deal out of this," he said gruffly, returning to his plate stacked with cheesecake and pie that he had pilfered from my roommate's wedding buffet. I was a bridesmaid. He was not invited. My roommate hated him. Which was probably why he had made an effort to show up. I doubt he would have come if I had asked him to.

"What you did last night," I stammered. "It was . . . " I didn't know what it was. I didn't even have the words to talk about it then. Later I would call it the worst night of my life. That day—the Day After—I rubbed my fresh bruises that would not be entirely hid, even under all the makeup I'd caked on them and finished, "It wasn't right."

He shrugged. "It's not what you think it was."

"What was it?" I pleaded, honestly wanting him to answer the question for me. How could I not know what had happened to me? *Tell me.*

"It was nothing. Just a mistake we made."

I knew enough to know that was not the right answer. The only mistake I had made was falling asleep. My mind latched on to the only tangible piece of evidence I had. "You ripped my bra!" It sounded so silly and dramatic when I said it aloud like that, and yet it was the one thing I kept coming back to. It hadn't felt violent when it was happening, and yet hours later as I sat on my floor numb and shaking, I kept twisting that bra over and over again in my hands and staring at the damage. It was one of those white utilitarian numbers that girls wear when they do not mean for their undergarments to be seen. And yet the thick straps were stretched and torn until both were broken completely apart.

Some of my other clothing was damaged too, but it was the bra that bothered me most. Particularly since it was the only white bra I owned, and I needed it to wear under my cream bridesmaid's dress the next day. Another bridesmaid had helped me pin it together in the bathroom of the reception hall. It took six safety pins to make it wearable. And they were digging into my skin as we spoke. Later I would put that bra, replete with safety pins, in my box—the box of evidence I hid in case he ever made good on his promise to kill me.

"Oh, I'll buy you a new one," he laughed. "How much do you need?"

"I don't want any money from you." That's what I told him that day, and that is exactly what I told the court representative after his sentencing for my assault and the later, more horrific sexual assaults of two other girls.

"I'm sorry, honey, but the judge ordered him to pay reparations. It's part of his sentence." She mistook my silence for something else and continued, "Don't worry, he won't be mailing it to you directly. They'll just garnish it from his wages, and the Department of Corrections will send it to you."

"I don't want his money," I repeated flatly.

"Surely you have therapy bills," she said kindly but with an edge. I was taking up too much of her time with my obstinacy.

I gritted my teeth. She knew I did. She had personally arranged for me to see a therapist. And I'd saved all the receipts like she told me to. But I refused to give them up. There are a lot of reasons I didn't want him to pay for my therapy. First, I didn't want to think of my therapist as being on his payroll. Second, the payments—even in their sterility—still tied me to him. Every time he saw how much his check was garnished, would he think of me? Think to himself, "Heh, big therapy month for Charlotte. Glad to know I'm still giving her nightmares!"? No thank you.

Despite my protestations, the checks began to arrive, as the dictates of justice will not be thwarted—not for offenders and apparently not for their victims either. The universe demands proper penitence from me for my stupidity on the night in question. The letters became my own personal, government-sealed hell. PTSD on ecru stationery. Part of their torture is their randomness. Of course, I got nothing while he was in prison. The way I knew he was back on the outside was the arrival of the first check, surprising me on a bright, sunny day like a punch to the stomach. For several months I got large-ish checks that left me feeling like an underpaid prostitute, and then I got nothing for months. Sometimes the checks were big, but more often they are small—but always they are random.

The other problem is their starkness. Take this most recent check, for instance—$5.24 arrived after more than a year of nothing. A year of forgetting to be nervous when I checked my mailbox. A year of not hiding ecru envelopes and wadded security-coded papers only to accidentally stumble upon them months later. A year of peace. I started to wonder. Had he been out of work this whole time? Did that mean he had gone back to prison? What if he had done it again but nobody told me? Perhaps he'd finally gone crazy.

Maybe this was my cut of his gambling winnings. Maybe he was homeless, living out of his car again. Was I taking $5.24 out of a beggar's cup? And why was the amount so small? Was he working as a fruit picker? Was he unable to get a decent job because of his felony record? Were his problems, after all, my fault—just like he'd always claimed?

I never cash the checks. It's not that I don't intend to—as my sister pointed out, I could just donate the money to a women's charity—it's that I just can't stand to deal with them. To deal with him. I don't want to sign my name to the back of a piece of paper that has his name on the front. No matter what he said that night, what happened does not bind us together forever.

The supreme irony of all of this is that of the three victims who testified against him, I am the only one who explicitly refused money from him. And to this day, I am the only one to have ever received the checks. He couldn't resist getting in one more blow.

Conclusion: What I Learned after One Year of Trying Everything

How to do a perfect push-up. The magic formula for weight loss. Which is better—supersets or circuit training? How about supersets in circuits? Was Adderall really the reason Lindsay Lohan lost her freaking mind (and, if so, why Mel Gibson hasn't tried it yet)? The answer to life, the universe, and everything. (42? Really??) Frankly, it would be easier to tell you what I *didn't* learn during my year of Great Fitness Experiments than to neatly summarize all the life lessons handed to me every time I got knocked on my keister. And if having five kids has taught me anything, it's to always take the easy route when it's offered to you. (Second lesson my kids have taught me: If you shove a red pom-pom ball up your nose, it will not magically turn you into Rudolph, although it will make Mommy ask the ER admissions lady if they sell punch passes.)

Three Things I Still Haven't Learned:

1. When to stop. You might think that after a year of trying every workout I could and reading every health and fitness book I could get my sweaty, calloused hands on that I'd be ready to move on to a new passion. You might also think that Mariah Carey would've discovered by now that she has other wardrobe choices besides the mini dress. You'd be underestimating both of us. If anything, I've only fallen more in love with the world of health and fitness research (also known as 10,000 Ways to Torture Rodents). Three years later, I'm still doing a new Great Fitness Experiment every month—feel free to join in the fun on my blog www.thegreatfitnessexperiment.com—and still loving every minute of it. (Well, except for that minute of one-legged pistol squats. Those made me so sore that, for a week, every time I had to use the bathroom, I had to drop the last three inches to the toilet because my quads gave out.)

2. When to listen. People are fountains of advice. Some of it great—"Before you roll up your yoga mat, fold it in half so the dirty part stays on the outside." Some of it not so great – "They don't sell any of the really good supplements in stores anymore (stupid FDA!), but I know this great Web site. Oh sure, it says it's only for veterinary purposes, but if you use a little math..." But the best advice is the kind that tells me about the giver. Similar to bars, therapists' offices, and women's restrooms in fancy restaurants, gyms are strangely conducive to sharing (over-sharing in many cases) by relative strangers. Maybe it's all the blood rushing to people's muscles and away from their brains, or perhaps it's the skimpy clothing (it's just a hop-skip from camel toe to bikini waxing!), but whether I'm in the locker room or on the weight floor or just waiting for my beloved TurboKick class to start, people will offer up all kinds of intimate details. War stories to weddings, family deaths to family desserts—the only opportunities that I'm really sad I've missed are those where I've been so intent on my killer workout that I didn't take time to listen to what people were really telling me.

3. How to stop embarrassing myself. Whether it's snapping myself in the butt with a jump rope and splitting my pants open or answering the rhetorical questions that my boot camp instructor likes to throw out ("Twenty more squats! Are you feeling the burn yet?" "Oh, yes, indeed! Except it's only in my left butt cheek, not sure why that is . . ."), my penchant for doing embarrassing things has only increased over the past few years. Luckily, my ability to embrace public humiliation has increased as well. I thank my kids for that—it's hard to be embarrassed by accidentally hawking a loogie down your own tank top once you've had the experience of your child having diarrhea in the middle of the grocery store and then dragging his butt on the floor in an effort to mitigate the flow. (Best part of that last story? While I was trying to help him, his brother took advantage of my inattention to liberate some tubes of lipstick and go all *Harold and the Purple Crayon* in aisle 5.)

It turns out that in the end, while I didn't find what I set out looking for (my pre-childbearing body, which apparently has joined Sasquatch and the Loch Ness monster in the misty realm between history and fantasy), I discovered that there is a lot more to the pursuit of health than whether or not I can wear my old jeans.

I learned that I'm stronger than I think. I learned that even if I can't do something perfectly the first time, it's still worth trying. I learned that *Steel Magnolias* still makes me cry even when it's close-captioned on Lifetime and I'm trying to run ten miles on the treadmill and people are staring at me as I drip snot and sweat all over the equipment. (I've also learned that I can't watch *I Didn't Know I Was Pregnant* while running on the treadmill as that show will also make me cry—not out of sentiment but raw, animal fear. Seriously, this is not something you tell a woman who gets pregnant every time she washes her underwear and her husband's together.) I've learned that "healthy" isn't a zero-sum game and even my failures can be turned into wins. I've learned that more isn't always better and less doesn't always mean defeat. I've learned that I can still love people even after I've seen them sit naked on the locker room bench without putting a towel down first. And while I can't quite stop making myself care about the number on the scale (yet!), I've learned that people are so much more important than their bodies. And that I'm a person too.

And I thought I wasn't going to tell you what I've learned! I hope that you will tell me what you have learned from your experiences as well. The number-one best thing about doing my Experiments, writing this book, and running my blog is getting to share in your lives too. I don't know how I managed to find all the amazing, beautiful, big-hearted, helpful people on the Internet and none of the trolls, but my readers (whom I all count as dear friends now) have become one of the biggest blessings in my life. I am so grateful for every one of you who has taken the time to share your story with me, read my stories, correct me, give me a big reality check, or even just laugh silently along with me every morning.

I've learned that we're all in this together.